BEHAVIOR MANAGEMENT

CWLA Best Practice Guidelines

CHILD WELFARE LEAGUE OF AMERICA

WASHINGTON, DC

The Child Welfare League of America is the nation's oldest and largest membership-based child welfare organization. We are committed to engaging people everywhere in promoting the well-being of children, youth, and their families, and protecting every child from harm.

CHILD WELFARE LEAGUE OF AMERICA, INC.
Headquarters
440 First Street NW, Third Floor, Washington, DC 20001-2085
E-mail: books@cwla.org

CURRENT PRINTING (last digit)
10 9 8 7 6 5 4 3 2 1

Cover design by Jennifer Geanakos

Text design by Mary Flannery

Printed in the United States of America

ISBN # 0-87868-845-5

Library of Congress Cataloging-in-Publication Data

CWLA best practice guidelines : behavior management/Child Welfare League of America
    p. cm.
  Includes bibliographical references.
  ISBN 0-87868-845-5
    1. Social work with children—United States. 2. Social work with youth—United States. 3. Problem children—Behavior modification. 4. Problem youth—Behavior modification.
  Child Welfare League of America. National Task Force on Behavior Management.

  HV741 .C85 2001
  618.92'89—dc21

                                                        2001052676

CONTENTS

FOREWORD

The Child Welfare League of America's National Task Force on Behavior Management developed the following best practice guidelines. The guidelines were developed in a generic format to ensure that they could be used in all settings that serve children and youth who have challenging behaviors. These settings include child day care and school age child care, foster care, kinship care, juvenile justice, boot camps, residential care, psychiatric hospitals, shelter care, day treatment, public and private education, and in-home services. These guidelines were developed by the task force between August 28, 2000, and August 8, 2001.

The purpose of these guidelines is to provide licensing and regulatory agencies with an effective tool for formulating administrative policies and procedures for behavior management. In addition, CWLA will use the guidelines to assist in the development of new program standards and the revision of current program standards for child day care, foster care, kinship care, group care, and juvenile justice. The guidelines will be available to providers interested in improving program practice and services to children and youth. The guidelines should also prove useful to accrediting bodies in their revision of behavior management standards.

The guidelines represent the best thinking of professionals across program areas and were developed to provide guidance to the field. These guidelines are not intended to be detailed descriptions of behavior management approaches or techniques, nor are they designed to take the place of standards. In contrast, CWLA standards are more prescriptive in nature, defining those practices considered most desirable, and establishing clear goals for the continuing improvement of services to children and their families. The task force strongly recommends the use of the *Best Practice Guidelines for Behavior Management* in the development or revision of behavior management programs and practice.

Lloyd Bullard
Director of Residential Care, CWLA

Introduction

The Child Welfare League of America is a national membership organization of more than 1,150 child-serving agencies throughout North America. Both public and voluntary agency members serve children, youth, and families in need of pregnancy services, parenting skills, adoption, foster care, kinship care, mental health treatment, substance abuse treatment, child day care, housing, independent living, residential group care, and juvenile justice services, as well as other essential supports and services. CWLA member agencies, service providers, foster parents, and caregivers are responsible for managing the behavior of troubled and needy children and youth in their care while ensuring their safety during periods of crisis intervention.

CWLA has long been concerned with the need for a broad array of tools and skills to deal effectively with children and adolescents who present challenging behaviors. Providers have traditionally expected states, accrediting bodies, and standard-setting bodies to furnish them with direction and guidance. The League, in an effort to address these concerns, has worked with states over the years on the revision and development of behavior management licensing rules and regulations.

Behavior management continues to be a complex issue. While providers are struggling to find more effective tools for managing the behavior of children and youth, they are also faced with the task of recruiting and retaining staff. The Bureau of Labor reports that demand for staff will rise during the next ten years, and the labor pool will continue to shrink significantly. Shortages will be especially visible in the areas of direct care staff, social workers, and support and administrative staff.

The growing crisis of staff shortages in child welfare can be seen in three areas. First, there is an insufficient number of qualified personnel to fill agencies' vacant positions. Secondly, when qualified staff members are found, many child welfare agencies are unable to compete with other industries' salaries and benefits. Lastly, once qualified staff are hired and trained, agencies are unable to retain them. Many agencies are experiencing high vacancy rates. Staff vacancy and turnover affect the consistency and quality of treatment, and can impact the safety of the children and youth being served.

To ensure that caregivers can successfully manage the increasingly difficult behaviors presented by children receiving service, providers must use two parallel approaches. The first is to develop effective behavior management tools. The second is to develop a comprehensive long-term staffing strategy that addresses issues of recruitment, retention, professional and career development, and establishment of competitive salaries and benefit packages. Only after the implementation of these strategies will providers be able to ensure that children and youth are kept safe during periods of crisis intervention.

In October of 1998, the *Hartford Courant* newspaper in Hartford, Connecticut, published a weeklong series demonstrating just how difficult it is for providers to manage behaviors of children and youth, and keep them free from injury and/or death. The *Hartford Courant* series produced a significant increase in the public awareness of deaths occurring in mental health and residential facilities during or shortly after the use of restraint or seclusion.

As a result of the increased public awareness of the risk of improper use of restraint and seclusion, numerous versions of legislation were proposed in several states and in the U.S. Congress. Additionally, the General Accounting Office filed a report, and the Department of Health and Human Services (HHS) proposed regulations regarding restraints and seclusion.

On October 19, 2000, President Clinton signed into law the Children's Health Act of 2000. The Act reauthorized the Substance Abuse and Mental Health Services Administration (SAMHSA), which established requirements regarding the use of restraints and seclusion in certain facilities. Two sections were written to address the use of these techniques in certain facilities. Part H applies to "a public or private general hospital, nursing facility, intermediate care facility, or other health care facility that receives support in any form from any program supported in whole or in part with funds appropriated to any federal department or agency." Part I applies to "nonmedical community-based facilities for children and youth." Several areas within the law require the HHS Secretary to develop regulations.

On January 22, 2001, Health Care Financing Administration (HCFA), renamed the Center for Medicaid and Medicare Services (CMS) announced its publication of the interim final rule with comment period for the use of restraint and seclusion in psychiatric residential treatment facilities that provide Medicaid's inpatient psychiatric services for individuals under age 21. The rule established a definition of "psychiatric residential treatment facility" as a facility that is not a hospital, but that may furnish such services. In addition, the rule sets forth a Condition of Participation (COP) stating that psychiatric residential facilities that are not hospitals must begin to provide, or continue to provide, the Medicaid inpatient psychiatric services benefit to individuals under age 21.

HCFA went beyond the language included in the Children's Health Act to provide greater protections regarding the use of restraints and seclusion than the law specified. The rule was scheduled to become effective 60 days after the publication date. President Bush, however, signed an executive order postponing the effective date to allow the new administration an opportunity to review the regulations.

On May 22, 2001, CMS published an amended interim final rule for the use of restraints and seclusion in psychiatric residential treatment facilities that provide Medicaid's inpatient psychiatric services for individuals under age 21. The amended rule addresses the concerns submitted in comments on the original interim final rule (January 22, 2001) by further clarifying which facilities are affected by the rule, revising the reporting requirements, clarifying the definition of "personal restraint," and broadening the personnel requirements for those permitted to order restraint and seclusion, accept verbal orders, and assess the physical and psychological well-being of residents.

Additionally, the amended rule requires any use of restraints and seclusion in a covered Medicaid psychiatric facility to be performed only upon an order and under the supervision of a physician, a registered nurse, or other licensed practitioner permitted by the state and facility to issue orders. CMS made these requirements consistent with those in the Children's Health Act of 2000, which mandates that restraints and seclusion may be applied only by properly trained staff. Furthermore, the amended rule addressed concerns regarding the shortage of registered nurses and board-certified psychiatrists. The amended interim final rule took effect immediately, May 22, 2001.

In the context of this national discussion regarding behavior management in child and youth care settings, and in an effort to address the need to care safely and appropriately for children and youth, CWLA set out to develop best practice behavior management guidelines. CWLA formed the National Task Force on Behavior Management on August 28, 2000. The task force included 35 representatives of advocacy groups, consumer groups, CWLA's member agencies, accrediting bodies, public and private agencies, national organizations, behavior management training organizations, medical professionals, attorneys, and others with expertise in residential group care, foster care, child day care, and juvenile justice. In addition, CWLA staff members participated in the development of the guidelines, providing support and assistance to the process (see Appendices).

The first task force meeting occurred in Washington, D.C., on November 1, 2000. The task force subcommittees developed the content for the following chapters: "Ethical & Legal Framework," "Administration and Leadership," "Continuum of Interventions," "Professional Development and Support for Staff and Caregivers," and "Medical Issues." The task force met again to develop further the draft guidelines on March 6, 2001, during the Child Welfare League's National Conference. Other national organizations and individuals, not represented on the task force, were given the opportunity to submit comments in response to the initial draft of the guidelines. Between April and June 2001, the CWLA Review Committee integrated comments and revised the guidelines. The Task Force was given another opportunity to comment on the revised draft in July, and the CWLA Review Committee made final revisions to the guidelines. The task force presented the final draft for publication on August 8, 2001.

CHAPTER 1

Ethical and Legal Framework

Introduction

Any discussion of behavior management practices should identify the prevailing laws and regulations that guide the use of nonphysical and physical interventions. Equally important is the identification of the ethical foundations that guide professionals' attitudes and practices in behavior management. In addition, we need to discuss basic rights that should be granted to children and families, and the responsibilities of every caregiver, provider, or organization using behavior management techniques.

It is not possible to list here all existing laws and regulations concerning behavior management, but it is possible to identify the legal, ethical, and general child and family principles that guide the discussion of behavior management across the continuum of services. To best address these principles, this chapter includes three separate and equally important sections:

- "Ethical Considerations" identifies the ethical precepts that should guide the use of behavior management techniques;

- "Rights of Children and Families" identifies the rights that should be granted to children and their families with regard to behavior management. This section also identifies, across disciplines, the guiding principles that define the rights of children and families;

- "Legal and Regulatory Considerations" describes the laws and regulations directing the use of behavior management techniques across the spectrum of services. In addition, this section builds upon the discussion of ethical considerations and the rights of children and families in order to recommend the best legal and regulatory practices for behavior management for all providers serving children and youth.

Ethical Considerations

Providers today have powerful means of controlling the individuals they serve. A variety of tools are available to providers to keep children and caregivers safe. These tools include verbal deescalation techniques; time-out; physical, mechanical, and chemical restraints; and seclusion. When used inappropriately, however, these tools of safety and security can become weapons of power and control. It is therefore essential that these practices operate within a clear ethical framework.

Ethics, by definition, is "a discipline dealing with good and evil and with moral duty, moral principles, or practice." It is the duty of each provider to ensure that the persons served are treated with respect, and that the environment is free from verbal and physical abuse and neglect.

Ethics from the Start

Regardless of the type of program or service provided, each provider should have a policy and procedures manual that includes the provider's written ethical standards or code of ethics. Ethical standards should cover the provider's mission and philosophy, the services provided and persons served, the family's role, and the responsibilities of caregivers for carrying out the program mission and vision. The standards should govern the proper treatment of individuals in the care of the provider and should touch every facet of the provider's program and processes.

Having ethical standards in place from the start will help to ensure that all caregivers understand what is expected of them and the consequences for not performing in an ethical manner. Information on ethical standards should be communicated clearly to prospective caregivers during the interviewing process to ensure that the caregivers are willing and capable of carrying out the mission of the program. Orientation and in-service training present additional opportunities to reinforce the provider's ethical standards. (See Chapter 5, Professional Development, for further information about training.)

Setting a Framework for Ethical Practice

Provider policy should require all caregivers to be adequately trained in the proper use of techniques for avoiding restraint, and the appropriate techniques to use when restraint and seclusion are necessary to keep an individual from hurting himself/herself or others.

Provider policy and procedure should convey that *restraint and seclusion may be used only on an emergency basis* when other less restrictive interventions have been or would be ineffective in averting danger to the individual or others. Restraint and seclusion must not be used as retribution or for convenience of caregivers, as a substitute for the individual's service plan, or in a way that interferes with the individual's service plan.

Ethical standards should require:

- development of individualized service plans that require use of the least restrictive and/or intrusive methods possible, and emphasize systematic application of learning principles with the intent of eliminating undesirable behavior;

- declaration that under no circumstances will the health and welfare of individuals be compromised; and

- compliance with all applicable federal, state, and local laws, and regulatory requirements.

The Rights of Children and Families

Wherever they are served, children and youth should have the following rights:

- to be served under humane conditions with respect for their dignity and privacy;

- to receive services that promote their growth and development;

- to receive culturally competent and linguistically appropriate services;

- to receive services in the least restrictive and most appropriate environment;

- to receive written information about the provider's policies and procedures, including a description of behavior management practices;

- to be served with respect for confidentiality;
- to be involved, as appropriate to age, development and ability, in assessment and service planning;
- to be free from harm by caregivers or others, and from unnecessary or excessive use of seclusion and restraint;
- to file complaints and grievances.

Families and guardians should have the following rights:

- to receive written information about the provider's policies and procedures;
- to receive services with respect for confidentiality;
- to be involved in assessment and service planning;
- to give and to withhold informed consent;
- to be notified following any use of seclusion or restraint, suicide attempt or completed suicide, medical emergencies, or any other seminal event in the life of their child; and
- to file complaints and grievances.

Informed Consent

Informed consent is a process of mutual understanding between the recipient of service and the service provider. Informed consent may be given only when an individual receives a clear, concise, written explanation that includes:

- the reason for the proposed intervention;
- an accurate description of the proposed intervention, including any specific techniques to be used;
- the potential benefits, risks, and side effects if the proposed intervention is used;
- the potential risks and benefits if the intervention is not used, including any service consequences;
- any exceptions to confidentiality;
- the likelihood of success of the intervention; and
- any possible alternative interventions.

Children and their families must have ready access to the provider's policies and procedures regarding their rights. The process of informed consent should include enough time and information for the child and family to make fully considered decisions. Although legal guardians have decision-making authority, every effort should be made to involve children and youth in service decisions. According to the American Academy of Pediatrics (AAP), children and young people should participate in decisionmaking regarding their care, commensurate with their development, and should provide assent whenever reasonable. Parents and physicians, as well as other service providers, should never exclude children and youth from the decisionmaking process unless there are persuasive reasons to do so (AAP, 1995).

Legal guardians have the right to refuse to consent to services and treatment. A provider may decide that a child or youth cannot be served as a result of refusal to consent. If there is such potential, the provider should include a discussion of all possible ramifications during the informed consent explanation of potential risks and benefits. Caregivers, providers, and organizations should comply with state laws regarding involuntary treatment.

Confidentiality

All parties have the right to confidentiality of medical and mental health services and records, except when laws or ethics dictate otherwise. Medical and mental health records should be treated as confidential and excluded from the records released routinely to school officials and other authorities. Any disclosures must be made with the informed consent of the family, and the informed consent of the youth if appropriate.

Grievances

Children, youth, and families have the right to assert grievances, to have grievances considered in a fair, timely, and impartial manner, and to exercise this right without fear of reprisal.

A grievance procedure should be a clear, written statement that includes:

- the procedure used to report complaints or grievances, including timelines;

- a confidential means for reporting alleged incidents of abuse by a caregiver;

- assurance that the complaint may be submitted to someone other than the caregiver named in the complaint;

- an opportunity for the child or youth to present his or her version of events and to present witnesses;

- a process for informing the complainant of the results; and

- a process for appeal.

Legal and Regulatory Considerations

The guiding principles for a legal and regulatory framework for the use of physical restraint and seclusion come from an examination of the U.S. Constitution and relevant Supreme Court cases that interpret it. The Court ruled in *Youngberg v. Ohio*, based upon prior holdings in *Estelle v. Gamble, Bell v. Wolfish,* and *Poe v. Ullman* that when a state takes someone into custody and holds him/her against his/her will, there is an "unquestioned duty to provide reasonable safety for all residents and personnel." The Court also recognized in the Fourteenth Amendment's due process clause a liberty interest of the individual to be free from bodily restraint, which needs to be balanced against the custodian's obligation to keep the individual safe from himself/herself or others. The standard set by the Court in *Youngberg* is that a resident cannot be restrained except when professional judgment deems it necessary to ensure safety.

Even though *Youngberg* involved a person in a nonvoluntary setting, the need to balance the duty to protect and the liberty interest to be free from bodily restraint as espoused by the Court surely applies to all service settings. Across all settings, sound professional judgment of caregivers is required to decide properly between these often-competing obligations.

State laws provide the legal authority for the regulation and licensing of child serving providers. Statutes authorize the promulgation of licensing standards, often referred to as regulations, rules, or requirements, which must be met for the state to grant permission to operate. Some licensing statutes specifically delineate the areas to be included in the licensing standards, and others do not.

Federal laws and some state licensing regulations establish the criteria to be met in the development of behavior management programs. It is important for each provider to be knowledgeable of the applicable federal and state laws as well as the applicable licensing regulations. Caregivers should be trained in these areas to ensure compliance.

Summary

This chapter identifies the central and crucial components of legal and regulatory considerations, ethical considerations, and the rights that should be afforded to children and their families when examining the issues of behavior management. These principles should serve as the foundation for the remaining chapters of the *CWLA Best Practices Guidelines for Behavior Management*.

CHAPTER 2

Administration and Leadership

Introduction

A provider's leadership and administration should provide the necessary structure, support, resources, and accountability to manage safely the inappropriate and potentially dangerous behavior exhibited by children and youth in care. Formulation of policies and procedures should be made in partnership with representatives of the communities to be served and with the input of experts in child discipline, behavior management, and restraint and seclusion. Licensing and certification of programs and individuals, likewise, should occur under a system of standards developed in collaboration with individuals who represent a wide range of perspectives and expertise regarding children and adolescents.

This chapter provides, from an administrative perspective, best practices concerning implementation and maintenance of a comprehensive behavior management system. It will address the following areas:

System-Wide Administration

- Placement and contract policy
- Licensing regulations
- External monitoring of providers
- Training of licensing and oversight professionals
- Incident reporting
- Advocacy and public awareness

Provider Leadership

- Creating a culture of safety and respect
- Consistency of practice with mission and goals
- Continuous quality improvement

- Role of governing and advisory boards
- Board awareness of best practice in behavior management
- Accountability and reporting to the board
- Board's role in policy and procedures
- Policies and procedures
- Responsibility for appropriate resources (quantity and quality)
- Credentialed workforce (training, supervision, and orientation)
- Strategic connections

System-Wide Administration

Parents, school systems, child welfare and mental health agencies, and the courts place children in a variety of settings in accordance with local and state laws. The systems responsible for child placement and for monitoring child service providers should ensure, first and foremost, that policies are in place to promote prosocial behavior. A secondary focus should be on the policies that providers follow and the techniques they use to manage children's behavior.

Community leaders and members should serve as advocates for children and for excellence in programming for children's needs. Professionalism in the care of children should be promoted, as well as adequacy of compensation for the care provided.

Placement and Contract Policy

Intake

Policies and practices should reflect concern for and appreciation of each child's unique needs. Except for detention settings, providers should not be mandated to adopt "no reject, no eject" policies. Instead, careful preplacement evaluation of the provider's ability to meet the child's needs should characterize the intake process. Providers should establish clear criteria for admission and should evaluate each applicant for service against those criteria. The child's routine and special needs and the provider's ability to meet those needs should be considered during the selection of a potential service provider.

Except in detention situations when intake and admission may be simultaneous, the intake process should be prior to admission and should afford the child and his or her family sufficient time to consider fully the service options and alternatives.

The intake process should include:

- an assessment of the child's needs in comparison to the services provided;

- an opportunity for the child and the child's parent or guardian to visit and meet with caregivers;

- an opportunity for the child and his or her parent/guardian to tour all areas where the child may receive services, including classrooms, recreation areas, living spaces, bedrooms, kitchen, and dining areas;

- an explanation to the child and parent or guardian of the rules and expectations of the provider, as well as behavior management practices used;

- an opportunity to view time-out rooms and quiet rooms; and

- an explanation to the child and family of the process for intake and admission decisions.

Admission

The person responsible for the child should accompany the child to the service setting, remain with him or her for a time, and keep in regular contact following admission.

At admission,

- the child and family should be taken on a tour of the facility;

- the child and family should be introduced to peers and caregivers; and

- the child should be given an opportunity to become familiar with the facility and with his or her personal space. If the provider is a day setting, that may include a cubby or locker and a desk or work area. If the setting is residential, the child should be taken to his or her bedroom and encouraged to unpack and get settled.

The child and family should be given the following information at admission, if it has not already been provided:

- a written description of the provider's rules and behavior management practices;
- a demonstration of the restraint procedures used by the provider;
- the provider's written complaint and appeal procedure.

Support Services

Providers should have at their disposal an array of services to assist them in promoting positive behavior in children and in dealing with challenging behaviors. Such "wrap-around" services should include individual and group counseling by qualified therapists, on-site, one-on-one attention through such programs as Foster Grandparents or Big Brother/Big Sister, and respite for caregivers from childcare responsibilities.

Providers and placing agencies should have sufficient financial resources to provide the child with "extras" such as field trips, and equipment for sports or community group involvement that are needed while the child is receiving services.

Contracts and Agreements

Contracts between providers and placing agencies should delineate clearly what each will provide, what the performance expectations are, how performance is measured, and what the consequences for nonperformance are.

Placing agencies should frequently monitor the provider via

- on-site visits with the child,
- review of provider records and policies,
- contact with individuals responsible for children's care, and
- review of regulatory history.

Agreements with parents should define clearly the expectations for parents and providers.

Licensing Regulations

Ensuring minimum acceptable standards for care of children outside the home is a public responsibility and influences the behavior of children in these care settings. The state or community should require all programs that accept children for care to be licensed or certified by a government-authorized entity as having met minimum standards for the type of care offered.

Licensing regulations should be developed through a public process in which the concerns of those affected as well as those of knowledgeable experts are actively sought by the regulatory body. A policymaking body should develop regulations that address child development, mental and physical health issues, the physical environment, services to be delivered, effectiveness of service delivery, encouraged and prohibited practices, safety issues, and consequences for violation of regulations. Regulations should ban any policy that denies access to the facility by the monitoring agency or that denies immediate access to the child or youth by the person or agency legally responsible for him or her. In the case of children and youth in custody of child welfare agencies or detention facilities, regulations should specify processes for notifying and responding to parents.

Regulations should set forth minimum training and experience requirements for staff of licensed providers. The requirements should delineate specific areas of training needed and number of hours needed in each area. Orientation and in-service training of caregivers should be mandated. All caregivers should be required to receive training appropriate to their positions and level of contact with children. Regulations should establish requirements for criminal background checks for caregivers.

Regulations should require licensed providers to report to them any critical incidents involving restraint or seclusion that result in serious injury to children or caregivers. Regulations should also require periodic reporting of aggregate provider data regarding restraints and seclusion. Regulatory agencies should establish guidelines for the collection, review, and utilization of restraint and seclusion data.

Regulations developed under this process should have the force of law. Communities should consider adopting a range of sanctions for violation of regulations, in addition to suspension or revocation of licenses.

The regulatory authority should establish an appeal process to allow licensees an impartial forum in which to contest actions taken against them.

External Monitoring

External monitoring promotes compliance with regulations and provides an opportunity to offer assistance before and after problems arise.

Monitoring done by the regulatory agency should include examination of the physical plant, family involvement in the program, caregiver interaction with children in care, activities the children are engaged in, proactive and reactive strategies the provider has employed, appearance of children in care, food service (if applicable), and compliance with previously cited regulations.

Regulatory agencies should inspect the provider annually, and preferably quarterly, at random times appropriate to its hours of operation. Annual fire, health, and safety inspections should be incorporated into the regulator's inspection regimen. Some inspections should be unannounced.

Agencies holding custody of children should conduct frequent on-site visits and should visit with the child alone, with caregivers alone, and with the child and caregiver together. Agencies should generally make unannounced visits in order to derive a more realistic picture of the child's experience in the setting.

Unless contraindicated in the child's service plan, family should visit the provider and observe the program in operation. They should be permitted to do so as unobtrusively as possible, even if their visit is unannounced. Parents should be encouraged and supported in participating in provider activities. Parents of children in school and day care settings should routinely observe when they drop off or pick up the child.

Complaints about the provider should be investigated by the regulatory agency and others, as appropriate (such as law enforcement if a crime is alleged, or the child protection agency if child abuse or neglect is alleged). Investigations should involve face-to-face contact with the alleged victim(s) and any witnesses, and should usually involve on-site contact with the caregivers. Whenever feasible, written statements from those who have knowledge of the event should be obtained. Provision for consultation with experts in relevant disciplines should be part of the investigation process, as needed.

Regulatory agencies and entities legally responsible for the child or youth should note if the provider has a history of taking frequent disciplinary actions with children in general or with a particular child. Such actions may indicate that the provider has accepted an individual it is unable to serve effectively.

The system should empower caregivers to report incidents and practices that they perceive as harmful to children and youth. Caregivers making such reports should be assured confidentiality.

Training for Licensing and Oversight Professionals

Licensing professionals, persons who investigate restraint and seclusion related incidents, and provider staff members who approve use of restrictive interventions should have knowledge and skills appropriate to their oversight responsibilities. It is recommended that these staff members receive, at minimum, training in behavior management equivalent to that provided to caregivers and supervisors working in the settings for which they have oversight responsibilities.

Incident Reporting

In order for monitoring to be effective and responsive, regulatory agencies and entities responsible for children must have timely notice of events that impact children and their behavior. Critical incidents involving restraint and seclusion that result in injury to a child or caregiver should be reported in writing to the regulatory agency by the end of the next business day. Such critical incidents should be reported to the person legally responsible for the child as soon as possible, and no later than within 24 hours. In nonresidential programs, such incidents should be reported as soon as possible, and no later than the end of the child's day.

Critical incident reports should include:

- a description of what happened;

- date and time of occurrence;

- intervention used, reasons for use, and the duration of the intervention;

- children involved;

- caregivers or others involved, including full names, titles, and relationship to the child;

- witnesses to the incident;

- person making the report;

- any injury to the child, including body chart or photo of any injuries;

- action taken by the provider;

- preventive actions to be taken in the future;

- any follow-up required; and

- documentation of supervisory or administrative review.

Incidents of serious injury during restraint or seclusion should be reported immediately to the parent or guardian of the child.

Suspected criminal activity by a child or youth or by a caregiver should be reported immediately to the appropriate law enforcement agency. Criminal activity should be reported to the regulatory agency by no later than the end of the next business day after such activity is identified.

Advocacy and Public Awareness

The provider's leadership must work actively to establish an advocacy position that draws attention and resources to the critical issue of vulnerable children. As policymakers and legislators are growing increasingly concerned about escalating levels of violence exhibited by young children, the tendency is to react with punitive measures. Children's advocates and child welfare leaders must find a common agenda to enable all to join in promoting proactive, developmentally appropriate responses to this escalating crisis.

It is imperative that child-serving agencies collect and disseminate valid data that will support the agenda of prevention and treatment in all levels of care.

Leadership must present a case that is based on successful outcomes instead of relying solely on anecdotal data. Advocates need to speak with one voice and understand the full continuum of care for children in order to be effective in promoting the agenda for at-risk children. The task is challenging because some taxpayers and legislators do not look favorably on children whose behaviors necessitate restraint. Leaders in organizations must provide caregivers with the tools and language to advance the agenda on behalf of children in care.

To be effective in influencing public policy and regulation, the public must be educated about the needs of behaviorally challenged children and youth. A campaign that celebrates successes and succinctly describes the causal factors can mitigate the myths and fears that drive punitive policy. Leadership should work on the local and state levels to forward this agenda for children.

Provider Leadership

A provider's leadership is responsible for developing, implementing, and maintaining a comprehensive behavior management system designed to prevent and safely manage inappropriate and potentially dangerous behavior. The level of effectiveness of any organization, in this regard, depends on the leaders' commitment to a well-designed and articulated behavior management system that is consistent with the organization's mission and philosophy. The leaders should be fully familiar with the behavior management system and understand its ethical and philosophical foundations and the core elements that are fundamental to its implementation and maintenance. There should be clear written policies, procedures, and guidelines that are communicated to all caregivers. Every caregiver should know what developmentally appropriate practice to use when confronted with potential crisis situations, and how to prevent, deescalate, and contain a child's difficult behavior.

Creating a Culture of Safety and Respect

- The provider's leaders should create an ongoing organizational culture of safety and respect. This begins with establishing a supportive work environment in which caregivers, children, and their families are valued and treated with respect. There should be an emphasis on safety.

- Incidents of restraint or seclusion involving injury to caregivers or children should receive *immediate* administrative review.

- All incidents of restraint or seclusion should receive administrative review.

- Policies and procedures should clearly prohibit corporal punishment and should establish safeguards against abusive practices.

- Caregivers should be well trained in the use of appropriate and proactive behavioral management techniques.

- Leaders should provide sufficient resources, including an adequate number of qualified caregivers.

- The leadership should support regular external and internal monitoring.

- Leaders should promote an organizational culture that values developmentally appropriate and therapeutic practice above control and expediency.

Leaders should take prompt and definitive action when concerns are raised about the safety and care of children.

Consistency of Practice with Mission and Goals

The provider's behavior management system should be consistent with the organization's mission, philosophy, and goals. The organization should have a clearly defined mission that is written and communicated to all staff members. Written behavior management policies and procedures should be consistent with the organization's mission and purpose. The provider's leaders and staff should periodically review the mission statement and policies and procedures to ensure that they continue to meet the needs of the children who are being served. These policies and procedures should clearly define safe practice and provide caregivers with the necessary guidelines and structure to ensure quality of care and supervision for children. Caregivers, the children or youth served, and their families should be involved in the development and ongoing review and revisions of the mission statement.

Continuous Quality Improvement

Providers should develop mechanisms for quality improvement that are appropriate to their size, mission, and services. A provider committed to ensuring delivery of quality services will establish processes for monitoring performance, reviewing policies and procedures, evaluating services, documenting and examining outcomes, and utilizing the results to make improvements in operation.

If the provider is a multilevel organization, the processes should involve individuals and groups at every level of the organization from individual caregivers to administrators and board members. The concepts central to continuous quality improvement, however, are also applicable to single-person and very small providers, as well as to "flat" organizations without multilevel structures.

Quality improvement processes may include external monitoring, contracting, and regulatory agencies. Any feedback received from agencies in response to critical incident reports, or as a result of licensing or monitoring activities, should be incorporated into the provider's quality improvement process.

Each provider should have a system for enforcing its documentation requirements. All required documentation of services provided, meetings, safety inspections, caregiver training and supervision, and outcome measures should be reviewed on a regular basis.

Each provider should establish systems for tracking the frequency, location, and type of critical incidents that occur. The data and management systems should have the potential to effectively monitor caregiver, child, and programmatic involvement in critical incidents. This documentation and monitoring system allows the provider to review incidents and make decisions about individual and organizational practice.

As appropriate to the provider's size and the needs of the children served, each provider should have access to clinical expertise and a multidisciplinary team. The clinician and/or team should review critical incidents according to established standards. The process should provide feedback to the provider's leadership and staff, including suggestions for prevention. Any situation that does not conform to established standards and protocols should require additional review and follow-up.

Because of the potential for abuse and liability in the use of restrictive behavior management procedures, it is strongly recommended that leaders and governing or advisory boards periodically engage external professional consultants to review behavior management policies, procedures, and provider practice. Such consultation can be secured from behavior management specialists with proper credentials or from national child welfare organizations. Consultation can also be secured through risk management firms, such as national liability underwriters. It is further recommended that any external consultation, and provider follow-up in response to such consultation, be appropriately documented in the provider records.

Providers and regulatory bodies should work to build strong interagency relationships to promote learning and improved practice. The provider and regulatory agencies share a common goal—to ensure the professional care and treatment of children and to safeguard client rights. If a provider or board member is aware of a potential problem in these areas, the provider should reach out to the licensing and regulatory bodies to invite their assistance in addressing and correcting such issues. Examples of problem areas include an unusually high frequency of restrictive treatment procedures, behavioral incidents that pose a risk to child or community safety, or a high number of client grievances related to behavior management practices.

Role of Governing and Advisory Boards

A provider that lacks a governing board of directors should establish an advisory board to review policies and procedures and to make recommendations about operational compliance with them. Boards of directors and advisory boards have a clear role and responsibility in assuring the safeguarding of client rights and the provision of effective care and treatment within the program. Boards also carry specific liabilities with regard to the use of restrictive treatment procedures that include the use of seclusion and physical restraint. Board members, therefore, should ensure that they are informed about these policies, practices, and incidents. Board members should further ensure that the provider has an adequate number of trained caregivers and that ongoing caregiver development programs are in place.

Board Awareness of Best Practice in Behavior Management

Board members have an obligation to be aware of legal issues, risks, and client rights relevant to the provider's behavior management practices. Provider administration and board leadership should provide orientation for new board members and ongoing education of all board members in these areas. This is particularly important when agencies use restrictive treatment procedures. Providers can build awareness through legal consultants, legal briefs summarizing new legislation, presentations from internal and external professionals, consultants, risk management experts, periodic journal articles, and review of national accreditation standards.

Accountability and Reporting to the Board

The board of directors employs and reviews the performance of the provider's chief executive officer. The board should ensure that written procedures developed by executives and staff members are consistent with board-approved policies. Policies and procedures should be reviewed periodically to ensure they are current with legal requirements and best practices.

Leaders should report to the board, at least annually, on the frequency and trends in provider use of restrictive interventions (including seclusion and physical restraint), and on injuries and client rights violations that may occur in the use of such procedures. Any incident involving the death or serious injury of a client should be reported to the board immediately. Any findings from licensing and monitoring agencies related to inappropriate procedures or use of restrictive behavior management should also be reported to the board. Board minutes should reflect the review of such information and any corrective action recommended or directed by the board.

Board's Role in Policies and Procedures

The board should ensure that written policies are in place to assure client safety, client rights, and the safeguarding of clients in behavior management and use of restrictive treatment procedures. The board should ensure that written procedures are consistent with the board-approved policies. The board should be sufficiently aware of the legal requirements and national best practice standards in this area in order to ensure that approved policies are consistent with such standards. Because of specific liabilities in the use of restrictive treatment procedures, it is also advisable for the board to seek review by legal experts in the process of developing these policies.

Policies and Procedures

Provider policies should address:

- Prohibited behavior management practices;
- Client rights and client safeguards in behavior management;
- Circumstances under which restrictive interventions may be utilized by caregivers, or policy prohibiting restrictive interventions;
- Documentation and reporting requirements in serious incidents;
- Abuse prevention and reporting requirements;
- Informed consent of parents and/or guardians in restrictive behavior management practices.

Procedures should include detailed instructions to personnel consistent with board-approved policies. The provider's behavior management principles and practices should be clearly stated. These procedures represent the "who, what, when, how" issues related to behavior management. Detailed procedures should be in place for any restrictive treatment procedure.

It is strongly recommended that agencies refer to national accreditation and best practice standards when developing and reviewing their own policies and procedures.

When agencies use restrictive interventions, written policy and procedure should define an administrative process to review all critical behavior incidents and restrictive procedures (incident by incident). This administrative review should evaluate whether the restrictive procedure was necessary, conducted according to defined provider standards, documented and reported as required, and whether follow-up corrective action is warranted.

Behavior management policies and procedures should be clearly communicated to all caregivers and supervisory personnel during preservice orientation and ongoing training. All personnel should be held accountable to these policies and procedures.

Responsibility for Appropriate Resources (Quantity and Quality)

Leaders should provide adequate resources, support, and professional development opportunities for personnel to ensure that they are able to provide quality services and support to the children. The safety and well-being of children is dependent on personnel having adequate training, supervision, and resources. These resources include:

- caregiver-to-child ratios necessary to adequately supervise and meet the needs of the children,

- supportive and ongoing clinical and front-line supervision,

- opportunities for staff development of strong and developmentally appropriate programming for the children,

- clearly written policies and procedures, and

- well-maintained equipment for activity programs.

Credentialed Workforce (Training, Supervision, and Orientation)

The provider's leaders should promote a comprehensive staff development program that includes an orientation program, core training as well as specialized training based on the population served, and crisis prevention and management training. A certified trainer who has completed a recognized and professionally developed training program should conduct crisis prevention and management training (including restraint and seclusion training). The course should be conducted according to recommended guidelines. Ongoing refresher training should be conducted with all caregivers according to recommended guidelines. At the completion of the original training and each refresher, caregivers should be expected to perform the skills at an acceptable level of performance. This performance should be documented, and staff should be held to a competency standard of performance in order to use restrictive treatment procedures.

Frequent and ongoing supportive supervision should be built into continuous monitoring of the behavior management system. Supervisors should be fully trained in all appropriate prevention, deescalation, and intervention techniques so that they can provide effective supervision, coaching, and monitoring. Supervisors should have reasonable expectations with realistic time frames and schedules for caregivers, so that they can accomplish tasks and respond to children's needs in a thoughtful and well-planned manner.

A postcrisis, multilevel response should be built into the practice. All children and caregivers should receive immediate support and debriefing following a crisis. Discussion of crisis incidents should be built into team/unit meetings so that all caregivers can learn from these situations.

(See Chapter 5, "Professional Development and Support for Staff and Caregivers," for comprehensive information about staff development and supervision.)

Strategic Connections

The provider's leadership should identify the external and internal resources necessary to implement and manage an effective response to the behavioral issues exhibited by the children and young people in their care. Each placing entity should identify the individuals and organizational influences that impact the life of each child. In their role as advocates, leaders may be required to establish new strategic alliances to ensure that the goals set forth in the child's treatment plan can be attained. Providers should respond to gaps in services that are identified by caregivers and that may necessitate building linkages with nontraditional partners such as law enforcement or business leaders.

Providers must work collaboratively with the various systems that may affect children in their care in order to avoid fragmented and diluted services. Managed care has resulted in an unprecedented shift in acuity of care, necessitating better transition planning and collaboration on all levels of the care continuum. Providers must work to positively influence policymakers, regulators, and administrative decisionmakers. These entities may be in child protection, juvenile justice, health care, mental health, child welfare, education, law enforcement, and executive and legislative branches on the local, state, and national levels. Providers must establish common language and goals as they promote and advance the agenda to ensure the safety and well-being of children and caregivers.

CHAPTER 3

Continuum of Intervention

Introduction

Behavior management includes a wide range of actions and interventions used in many different settings in which adults are responsible for the care and safety of children and youth. These settings include residential group care, family foster care, psychiatric hospitals, day treatment, child day care, in-home services, educational programs, shelter care, juvenile detention, school age childcare, and others. Behavior management includes a continuum of activities. On one end of the continuum would be proactive, preventive, and planned use of the environment; routines; and structure of the particular setting. On the other end would be less restrictive interventions such as positive reinforcement; verbal interventions; deescalation techniques; therapeutic activities; and loss of privileges. Behavior management also includes more restrictive interventions such as time-out; physical escorts; physical, chemical and mechanical restraints; and seclusion. These guidelines are intended to be applicable to all settings in which children who exhibit difficult behaviors are served. It is understood that certain interventions may be approved and utilized in some settings and prohibited in other settings.

Aggressive, assaultive, self-destructive, acting-out children and youth have the potential to cause harm to self or others. When adult caregivers attempt to prevent these same individuals from causing harm through the use of restraint and seclusion, these techniques create additional potential for harm, including serious injury and/or death. Any behavioral interventions used by caregivers must be premised on the goal of *"first, do no harm."* It must be acknowledged that the use of restraint and seclusion, even when necessary, are high-risk procedures that are inherently dangerous, and that there are no "fail-safe" techniques. *Although we may not know how to eliminate negative outcomes, we do know how to minimize them.*

Restraint and seclusion should be used only in an emergency, when there is an imminent risk of harm to the individual or others, and no less restrictive intervention has been or is likely to be effective in averting the danger. Because restrictive interventions have the potential to produce serious consequences (such as physical and psychological harm, loss of dignity, violation of an individual's rights, and even death), providers must continually explore ways to prevent, reduce, and eliminate their use. Nonphysical interventions should always be the first choice, unless safety issues demand an immediate physical response.

This chapter will provide best practice guidelines for a continuum of behavior management interventions. It addresses the following aspects of effective behavior management practice:

- Individualized service planning
- Selection or development of behavior intervention models
- Proactive and preventive planning
- Deescalation methods
- Physical interventions
- Debriefing, documentation, and follow-up

Individualized Service Planning for Behavior Management

Children and youth with behavioral difficulties that may necessitate the use of restraint or seclusion should have in their individualized service plans specific goals and objectives that address the targeted behavior(s) requiring the use of restraint and/or seclusion.

Service plans should be documented in the child's/youth's permanent record and should be communicated to all individuals responsible for providing supervision and care. Each plan should include:

- documentation of the participation of the parent, custodian, or guardian, and the child or youth (depending on the young person's age) in the development of the plan;
- written consent to the plan by the child or youth, if age-appropriate, and the parent, custodian, or guardian;

- a summary addressing prior intervention methods, documentation of the reasons the intervention failed, and the rationale for establishing new interventions;

- identification of targeted behavior(s);

- reason given to the child or youth for the implementation of the behavior management intervention;

- the criteria for removing the targeted behavior from the plan;

- a procedure for monitoring the correlation between a targeted behavior(s), behavior intervention, and outcomes;

- a review of the plan's effectiveness, to occur a minimum of every 30 days;

- a process to review and revise any plan that is determined to be ineffective or has demonstrated little to no progress;

- documentation of every restraint and seclusion in the child's/youth's clinical files; and

- assurance that all persons implementing the plan are trained and currently certified in behavior management.

Selection or Development of Behavior Intervention Models

Many providers are faced with the challenge of selecting or developing a behavior intervention model. One of the first steps should include a review of the provider's mission statement, which should embrace an overall goal for the children and youth served. This review process should not be limited to administrators, but should include all levels of staff. By clearly understanding the provider's mission and desired outcome for those served, the provider can develop a framework for achieving those outcomes. The provider must decide whether to develop its own model, or opt for one of the models currently available, such as the teaching-family model; guided group interaction; positive peer culture; point and level systems; positive youth development; risk and resilience; the caring profile; or one of numerous others. If the provider decides to choose one of the models currently available, it may be necessary to adapt the model to meet specific needs.

Whether the provider decides to use an existing model or develop its own, it is crucial that caregivers, clinicians, administrators, and any other staff members responsible for the supervision and care of the children and youth actively participate in the process. The success of any behavior model depends on the staff's investment. Staff ownership requires the full and equal participation of all staff members. It is extremely important to involve direct caregivers at the onset of this process, as they are the ones who spend the greatest amount of time with the children and/or youth and will be primarily responsible for the implementation of the model developed or selected.

A behavior model should be individualized and take into account the developmental stage of the child. It should not require that individuals conform to the model; rather, the model must be adaptable to the unique needs of the children being served. In addition, the behavior model must be as simple as possible. Any child or youth in the program should be able to understand and explain the model. The provider's leadership, culture, staff investment, population served, and method by which the behavior model is implemented determines how a behavior model functions within a particular setting.

Creating a developmentally appropriate behavior model for children and adolescents requires that providers develop programming that offers daily skills training, social skills training, challenging and meaningful activities that increase coping skills, and team cohesiveness. Staff members must be invested in providing children and youth with quality care; however, this is not enough. The provider must also invest in the staff, which means providing them with appropriate, quality training in communication, relationship building, behavior management, active listening, team building, and cultural diversity.

Proactive and Preventive Planning

Understanding Behavior, Crisis, and the Environment

The key word in this section of the guidelines is "understanding." A strong understanding or comprehension of positive interventions allows caregivers to transition confidently from knowledge to practice. Caregivers who are confident that they are receiving adequate training and support, opportunities for practice, refreshers, and proper supervision are more likely to perform safely and wisely. Child and youth-serving providers must be allowed adequate time to orient, train, and posttest staff in key areas before they have sole responsibility for children and youth. (See Chapter 5 for orientation and training information.)

Self-Management is the Goal

When conceptualizing positive behavior approaches for children and youth, the term behavior management is often used to describe what staff "do." To think of behavior management in this context is, however, a bit misleading. For behavior to be truly managed, the individuals must manage it themselves. Therefore, essential aspects in serving children include teaching, encouraging and enhancing the child's growth, and fostering development and self-management. This is, of course, easier said than done. Individuals who have been raised in positive family environments, with many supports, often struggle on a daily basis to manage their own behavior. For children and adolescents with complex and traumatic life experiences, this developmental task is even more complicated.

What then is at the core of helping children and youth to manage their own behaviors? At least three key ingredients appear to be necessary to develop and internalize these skills:

- A positive structured environment that focuses on growth and learning as opposed to controlling behavior,

- A focus on the relationship between the child or youth, and adults, and

- Quality educational and activity programming that promotes the achievement of developmental milestones for the child or youth.

A Positive, Structured Environment

The environment or milieu where children and youth play, work, and live has a powerful impact on their safety and well-being and is a critical driving force in their development of skills. The environment should contain ample space for the number of people served and should reflect a proactive program designed to minimize behavioral difficulties. The attitudes and beliefs of caregivers are as vital to creating a positive environment as the physical space itself.

The following environmental guidelines apply to spaces where children live, work, and play.

For all spaces:

- Respect personal space and belongings;
- Provide appropriate furnishings and equipment that are safe, clean, and well maintained;
- Eliminate visual "blind spots" and other impediments to observing and hearing children;
- Provide visual as well as verbal prompts (rules, expectations, schedules clearly posted);
- Attend to cultural diversity in displays of prints, posters, and other adornments that are reflective of the children and communities served;
- Create a sense of ownership and pride in the environment via chores, decorating contests, etc.

For living spaces:

- Encourage "personalization" of sleeping areas/bedrooms (toys, photos, and posters);
- Consider children's need for privacy;
- Attend to children and youth who show signs of anxiety at bedtime.

For classrooms:

- Create bright, colorful learning environments.
- Create "personal spaces" and "time-out" areas.
- Assess need for assigned or preferential seating.
- Plan culturally competent curricula.

For dining areas:

- Consider the effects of poverty and deprivation on children and youth (specifically, access to food and histories of food deprivation as punishment).

- Maintain visually pleasant, clean dining area with sufficient space for those served.

- Keep furniture, dinnerware, and utensils well maintained, and have motivational and nutritional visuals on walls.

- Set and communicate clear rules and expectations for mealtime routines and behaviors—entering and leaving the dining area, caregiver and child seating arrangements, caregiver role-modeling during meals, setting up and clearing of tables, number of diners away from tables at one time, mealtime conversation, sharing and passing food, and procedures for dismissal from the table and other interventions.

- Adhere to nutritional standards and posting of menus.

- Serve a variety of foods with consideration for cultural and ethnic diversity.

More restrictive vs. less restrictive environments. The population served in a given setting should determine the type of environment. For example, settings that serve juvenile offenders may require more aspects of a controlled milieu to serve children and youth effectively. In general, in a controlled setting caregivers are more likely to engage in controlling actions that may in turn lead to increased behavioral difficulties. The more caregivers seek to control, the more children and youth resist, and power struggles ensue. Power struggles are often the antecedent to restraint and seclusion.

No matter how restrictive a setting is, no caregiver should ever violate the rights of children to have food, shelter, and clothing, and to be treated with respect. A primary goal of every provider should be to make each child or youth feel safe and secure. (See Chapter 1 for more information about the rights of children and youth.)

A more restrictive environment may have the following qualities:

- Staff roles may be rigidly prescribed.
- There are numerous rules and procedures.
- There is a rigid schedule.
- The organization is hierarchical with rigid boundaries.
- Activities may be underutilized and are often earned.
- Children may have limited contact with people outside of the program.

In contrast, a less restrictive, but structured environment may have these attributes:

- There are rich and complex resources.
- A planned program includes some flexibility.
- There are well-defined group and individual goals.
- Experiences are challenging and interesting.
- There are rules and procedures for safety and efficiency.
- The organization has clear, multiple lines of communication.
- Activities are used to focus interest and are considered part of the treatment and education.
- There are open interactions with others outside of the program.

Relationship Between the Child or Youth and Caregivers

A key component in thc child or youth's success in developing the ability to manage his or her own behavior lies in the quality of the relationships developed with others in the environment, especially the adults. Children emulate what they observe and experience. When the relationships around them are trusting, caring, respectful relationships, children learn to trust, care, and respect. When children form trusting, caring relationships with caregivers, it may be their first experiences with positive relationships. The caregiver who is trusted and respected by a child will usually be more effective in behavior management than will a caregiver whose relationship with the child is less positive.

Providers should establish internal guidelines for relationships between caregivers and children and youth. All staff members should understand the provider's philosophy regarding caregiver roles and relationships with children. Any limitations should be clear to caregivers and children. Some providers encourage personal relationships and establish criteria for approving buddy, mentor, big brother, and visiting resource relationships between staff and children. Other providers prohibit contact between children and staff outside of the program and discourage personal relationships within the program. The biopsychosocial histories of children, their ages and needs, should influence the provider's development of such guidelines. For example, in a child care setting serving preschool children, affectionate physical contact between caregivers and children may be essential and desirable, while in a residential setting serving adolescents, physical contact between caregivers and youth may be prohibited. Each provider should establish clear guidelines about the expectations for relationship building between caregivers and children or youth, as well as policies and procedures that protect young people from abuse and inappropriate physical contact.

Quality Educational and Activity Programming

A significant aspect of engaging children or youth in managing their own behavior is that of quality activity programming. What happens on a daily basis in the child's life is critical to the achievement of developmental milestones. The types, frequency, and the depth of the therapeutic activities for young people in care are important to consider.

Appropriate activities may be the cornerstone of building an appropriate educational or therapeutic environment. They enhance the individual service planning for the child or youth and are supported by a multidisciplinary approach. Activities provide a focus and positive anticipation for both youth and caregivers.

The following principles apply to successful activity planning:

- The activity should activate.
- Structure precedes freedom.
- Knowledge and skill precede creativity.

- Many activities can be adapted to be appropriate for children and youth in any setting or age group.

- Process and product are both important.

- Clear and compelling goals for each activity help to focus peoples' energy productively.

- Behavior is best managed within and by an activity, rather than having an activity earned.

- When children are engaged in entertaining, productive, enjoyable planned activities, they are likely to develop the skills and abilities to engage in appropriate spontaneous activities.

The therapeutic activities that are most effective are varied and capture the interest of and meet the developmental needs of the children and adolescents served. Young people can be meaningfully involved in the planning and execution of the activities, thus allowing them to learn skills in planning, teamwork, and management of time and resources.

A balanced developmental activity program:

- reflects an overall positive valuing of activity;

- is considered a core of the program, not a "privilege" to be earned;

- utilizes caregivers' interests and enthusiasm;

- is directly derived from programmatic and individual service plans;

- provides guided exposure of children to *all* activity areas;

- allows some choice about participation;

- allows and encourages in-depth interest and further growth in one or a few areas;

- ties into developmental sequences of the activities themselves, of occupations, and of social, cognitive, physical, and emotional development;

- manages behavior *within* activities;

- provides sufficient activity to each child;

- is family centered or focused; and

- continues to build greater skill development.

Deescalation Methods

The formal meaning of the word "deescalate" is to decrease in intensity, magnitude, or amount. The purpose of "deescalation" as a behavior intervention is to engage with a potentially violent child in a manner that helps him or her to meet needs in ways that are not harmful to self or others. When deescalation is used appropriately, the goal is to intervene in such a way that the child or youth is able to exercise self-control and stop the escalation into violence.

There are many methods of deescalation that can be used to minimize the potential for violent behavior. Deescalation is an approach based on sound principles that can use a variety of frameworks for implementation. A number of methods can be effective, so long as they conform to the basic principles of respecting the rights of the child/youth, using the least restrictive method (matching the response to the level of injury threatened), and continuing efforts to coach the client into self-control, thus preserving his or her dignity.

It is important to note that interventions included in these guidelines do not represent any one model of behavior intervention, nor are they presented in a recommended sequence. All of these interventions may be helpful for some children some of the time.

Deescalation Methods and Guidelines

Deescalation methods and guidelines are outlined below.

- Assess and identify correctly the level of danger being presented by the child or youth to ensure that staff members do not overreact or under-react.

- Attempt to identify the motive for the child/youth's behavior, i.e., what need the child/youth is attempting to meet with the behavior. The intervening staff can work within the framework taught by the provider to identify and respond to children.

- In situations where a child/youth is either not yet threatening dangerous behavior, or is threatening only minor levels of danger, use verbal (or nonverbal) crisis intervention designed to provide a match for the motive expressed, or to specifically address the assessed reason for the behavior displayed.

- Place the caregiver in proximity to the child.

- Use positive touch.

- Provide *nonverbal* signals designed to help a child regain self-control, paying attention to posture, gestures, position, voice quality, speech content, and eye contact.

- Offer assistance to a child whose escalation may be due to frustration with, or inability to perform, a task.

- Take care to exercise self-control as an intervening caregiver (self-assessment—"How and what am I feeling right now?")

- Keep communication short and simple, and pay attention to tone and facial expression to be sure one can be heard and understood by a child or youth who is in a physiological crisis ("fight and flight") and thus dealing with reduced blood flow to the brain.

- Exercise patience and do *not* set a timeline in which a child or youth must regain self-control without use of more restrictive interventions.

- Remain spontaneous so that verbal interventions can be changed to match a changing set of motives on the part of the child.

- Remain culturally sensitive to verbal phrases and tones and physical (nonverbal) gestures and postures that might be misinterpreted by a child and thus provoke further escalation.

- Praise children who are doing well.

- Maintain consistency with other caregivers.

- Utilize additional staff or adult resources; switching out of power struggles can be helpful.

- Structure the environment to remove audiences, ensure the environment is danger free, and lower stimulation.

- Use reflective, supportive listening.

- Refrain from making reference to consequences. *Never threaten the use of restraint.*

- Use clinical assessment when appropriate to determine risk level.

Prompting

Prompts are nonthreatening and nonjudgmental. They should be delivered in a neutral and calm tone. Often, prompts are the initial intervention and can set the tone for the entire interaction between caregiver and child. Prompts can be used proactively to anticipate problems or give children advance notice of an impending change.

Redirection

In redirection, caregivers shift a child's attention from an undesirable or inappropriate activity or behavior to a more neutral or positive one. This can be accomplished by finding creative opportunities for positive outlets for children. Redirection often is extremely effective as a tool to help children on the verge of a tantrum to avoid serious consequences.

Planned Ignoring

Caregivers frequently employ this tool to stop harmless, nonthreatening, attention-seeking behaviors. Planned ignoring is a passive intervention and is not always effective. It is crucial for caregivers using this technique to assess situations carefully. It is important to determine whom else the child is engaging in the behavior. What effect is the behavior having on the group? What is the reason for the child's behavior?

Structuring the Environment

The caregiver should be constantly aware of where specific interventions take place and how the arrangement of the physical space can influence individual and group behavior. Caregivers should take into account such issues as space, volume, and cleanliness. The general philosophy is that a clean and orderly environment fosters a calm and therapeutic milieu.

Directive Statements

When other interventions have proved ineffective or when a behavior calls for a more direct approach, caregivers can use directive statements. Clearly communicated statements that inform children what to do are often effective.

Directions should be given clearly and said with meaning. Directive statements should sound authoritative and not be framed as requests. If possible, directive statements should be used only after other interventions have not resulted in the desired behavior.

Time-Out

For purposes of these Guidelines, the following definitions are used:

During **time-out** a child does not receive positive reinforcement and does not participate in the current routine or activity. The criteria for ending the time-out should be clear to the child.

During a **nonexclusionary time-out** the child does not participate in the activity and does not receive reinforcement, but is still able to observe others participating in the activity and receiving reinforcement.

An **exclusionary time-out** removes the child from an activity to a specified location where he or she is unable to participate, observe, or hear the activity.

Time-out is a valuable behavior management tool. It can be used to address any inappropriate or target behavior. All time-outs should be as quick as possible while allowing the child necessary time to regroup and focus. Appropriate staff ratios must be maintained for the group when a caregiver is supervising a time-out. When completed, the caregiver and child should process the behavior leading up to the time-out and should discuss alternatives before the child returns to the group or activity.

Time-out areas must be safe, well maintained, kept at an appropriate temperature, and an appropriate size to accommodate the child comfortably. A child in time-out must be observable at all times. A child or youth may not be placed in time-out behind a closed door unless a caregiver is present.

Special Considerations for Early Childhood and Young Children

As with other categories of care, there has been an enormous increase in the number of children in day care who exhibit difficult behaviors. Caregivers should use positive, developmentally appropriate methods of discipline and guidance that encourage self-control, self-direction, positive self-esteem, social responsibility, and cooperation. Prevention of behavioral problems should be emphasized by providing appropriate, educationally valuable materials and activities in an organized, stimulating environment. Set realistic expectations for young children when planning the program. For example, toddlers should not be expected to sit quietly through a 30-minute group activity. Children should be praised and encouraged for positive behavior; inappropriate behavior should be redirected or guided into more positive behavior.

Time-out, if used, should be used to supplement, not substitute other developmentally appropriate, positive guidance techniques. Time-out must be time limited, with approximately one minute for each year of a child's age. Time-out should occur immediately after the inappropriate behavior; otherwise the intervention is ineffective for producing the desired outcomes. Time-out should be used only until the child regains control. The caregivers must explain the reason for the time-out to the child in language he or she can understand. Preschoolers can be expected to understand time-out under adult supervision. School children who have begun to develop self-control and a sense of personal responsibility can understand the removal of privileges as consequences for undesirable behavior. When a child is removed from the group as a discipline measure, the child must remain under adult supervision at all times; children must never be left unattended behind closed doors.

When restraint is necessary for a child's self-protection or for the protection of others, it should be done by holding the child as gently as possible. The restraint should be stopped as soon as possible. Mechanical restraints should not be used to restrain young children. The decision to restrain a child should be made by the most experienced caregivers and only made in extreme circumstances. Persons who provide training for caregivers in the use of physical restraint must have extensive experience with young children and with physical restraint.

For children who have special needs, including behavioral and emotional disabilities, the provider should consult with professionals and family of the child to design appropriate and effective behavioral interventions.

As with older children, best practice requires that children be involved in the development of rules for setting behavioral limits appropriate for their age.

Physical Interventions

Challenging behaviors serve a purpose for the individuals who exhibit them. The central issue is defining the purpose of a particular behavior for that particular individual, and determining what intervention and behavior support is the "best practice" for that person. At times, that purpose may not be readily visible or apparent, but that does not change the fact that the behavior serves a purpose; it merely means that the purpose may not be known.

Physical interventions are, by nature, reactive responses rather than proactive. *Physical interventions should be used only in emergency circumstances and only to ensure the immediate physical safety of the individual or others when no other less restrictive intervention has been, or is likely to be, effective in averting the danger.* Physical interventions should be used only for the purpose of protection, and should not be used to change behavior in situations where the need for protection is not present. The safety of all individuals is paramount. Only the least restrictive intervention necessary to keep the child and others safe should be used. The use of physical intervention and restraint techniques must be individualized and should be terminated as soon as possible.

Definitions

Definitions of restraint techniques vary between experts and across jurisdictions, but conceptually the main types can be defined as follows:

Physical escort is the temporary touching or holding of the hand, wrist, arm, shoulder, or back for the purpose of inducing an individual who is acting out to walk to a safe location.

Physical restraint is the application of physical force by one or more individuals that reduces or restricts the ability of an individual to move his or her arms, legs, or head freely. Physical restraint does not include the temporary holding of an individual to assist him or her to participate in activities of daily living.

Mechanical restraint is the use of any physical device to limit movement and prevent harm to self or others. It does not include devices such as orthopedically prescribed devices, surgical dressings or bandages, protective helmets, or any other methods that involve the physical holding of a child for the purpose of conducting routine physical examinations, conducting tests, protecting the child from falling out of bed, or to permit the child to participate in activities without the risk of physical harm.

Chemical restraint is the use of any psychoactive medication as a restraint to control behavior or restrict the individual's freedom of movement that is not a standard treatment for the individual's medical or psychiatric condition.

Therapeutic hold is a physical restraint.

Seclusion is the placement of an individual in any room against his or her will, where the door is unable to be opened voluntarily by the individual, to prevent harm to self or others.

Throughout this section, guidelines will be presented that are intended to be appropriate in a wide range of settings in which restraint and/or seclusion are authorized and applied.

Guidelines

Initial Assessment and Admission

Any provider that uses restrictive behavior management interventions should complete a comprehensive assessment (as described in Chapter 4) during intake, before or at admission, and should provide parents and guardians with required written information and consents.

Caregiver Training and Certification

A provider that authorizes caregivers to use physical interventions must require them to complete appropriate orientation and training. (See Chapter 5 for information about staff development.)

Restraint

Use of Restraint

- A restraint may be used only in emergency circumstances and only to ensure the immediate physical safety of the individual or others when no other less restrictive intervention has been, or is likely to be, effective.

- Emergency circumstances are limited to those situations that endanger the physical safety of the individual or others.

- The restraint used must be the least restrictive intervention that is most likely to be effective in resolving the emergency.

- Any restraint must be limited to the least amount of time possible to address the situation and promote safety.

Prohibited Practices for Restraints or Seclusion

Restraints and seclusion should never be used

- as a threat of punishment or form of discipline,
- in lieu of adequate staffing,
- as a replacement for active treatment, or
- for caregiver convenience.

The following practices are prohibited:

- Pain compliance, slight discomfort, trigger points, pressure points, or any pain-inducing techniques (whether for brief or extended periods);

- Hyperextension of any part of the body (pushing or pulling of the knees, elbows, shoulders, limbs, joints, fingers, thumbs, or neck beyond normal limits);

- Putting the person at significant risk of hyperextension by placing any part of the person's body in a position that is beyond normal limits (i.e., holding one or both arms behind the back and applying pressure, pulling, or lifting);

- Joint or skin torsion (twisting or turning in opposite directions);

- Pressure or weight on chest, lungs, sternum, diaphragm, back, or abdomen, causing chest compression (i.e., positional or restraint associated asphyxiation);

- Straddling or sitting on any part of the body or any maneuver that puts pressure, weight, or leverage into or on the neck or throat, on any artery, or on the back of the person's head or neck, or otherwise obstructs or restricts circulation of blood or obstructs an airway;

- Any type of choking, hand chokes, arm chokes, sleeper hold; any type of neck or head hold where the head is used as a lever to control movement of other body parts, or any type of full or half nelson, or head lock;

- Any technique that involves pushing on the person's mouth, nose, eyes, or any part of the face, or covering the face or body;

- Any maneuver that involves punching, hitting, poking, pinching, or shoving.

Seclusion

The Child Welfare League of America recognizes that some states have historically depended on the use of seclusion and do not currently have other safe, available alternatives. However, every effort must be taken to elevate practice and keep children safe from abuse when in care. Seclusion must be used only with continuous visual monitoring, internal controls, and strong licensing and/or accreditation oversight.

Used appropriately, seclusion may prevent harm to the individual or to others in the immediate environment, and it may prevent transfer to a more restrictive setting (e.g. hospital, jail, etc.).

Used inappropriately, seclusion may further traumatize an individual, reinforce feelings of hopelessness and helplessness, and serve as a convenient and safe place to "park" difficult-to-manage individuals.

Use of Seclusion

- Seclusion should only be employed as a last resort to protect an individual from harming self or others.

- Seclusion must be part of a documented continuum of behavioral interventions.

- Unless contraindicated by the severity of the behavior, less restrictive behavioral interventions should always be employed prior to use of seclusion.

- Each and every use of seclusion must be documented and subsequently reviewed, in a timely manner, by the individual's clinical team.

- Seclusion should never be employed as a form of punishment, discipline, or for staff convenience.

- Seclusion should be promptly terminated when a client regains control.

Seclusion Rooms

Seclusion rooms must meet all applicable state and local fire and safety codes. Seclusion rooms must be designed specifically for the purpose and must be carefully assessed for safety before use. Seclusion rooms must be safe, clean, and well-maintained; must have adequate light and ventilation; and must maintain an appropriate room temperature.

Monitoring Individuals in Restraint or Seclusion (Observation)

- A trained observer should be present whenever possible to monitor the use of restrictive interventions. The designated staff should receive special training in the observation of all types of restraints and seclusion.

- Staff trained in the use of emergency interventions should be present.

- Staff monitoring the individual will be present in, or immediately outside, the seclusion room to ensure the safety of the individual.

- Monitor the resident's circulation, skin color, respiration, and range of motion. Refer to Chapter 4 for detailed guidelines for monitoring children and youth during restraint and seclusion.

- Video monitoring of an individual in seclusion may be used only if the caregiver is responsible for monitoring only one child or youth, and if the caregiver is located immediately outside the seclusion room. Video monitoring may not be used as a substitute for required periodic face-to-face monitoring.

- Any injuries requiring first aid and/or medical care sustained during a restrictive intervention should be reported to the person designated by the provider.

- The child or youth's parent or guardian should be notified immediately of any injuries requiring first aid and/or medical care sustained during restraint or seclusion.

Debriefing, Documentation, and Follow-Up

Debriefing

Supervisory staff should always review incidents in which behavior management techniques are utilized. Necessary debriefing should follow procedures outlined in agency policy and be supported by training in effective implementation. In addition, follow-up and debriefing can be viewed as part of the ongoing training process for caregivers.

- Within 24 hours after a resident has been restrained or secluded, the caregivers involved and the child or youth should participate in a face-to-face discussion.

- Discussion can also include other staff and the child or youth's parent(s) or legal guardian(s) when it is deemed appropriate by the provider.

- Discussion must be conducted in a language that is understood by the child and the family or guardian.

- Provide all parties an opportunity to discuss the circumstances that resulted in the use of restraint or seclusion, and strategies each could employ to prevent the need for restraint or seclusion.

- Include in the debriefing only those persons whose presence will not jeopardize the well-being of the child or youth.

- Hold a separate debriefing of staff involved in the emergency safety intervention, and a review by appropriate supervisory and administrative staff of the situation that required the use of restraint or seclusion. Focusing on positive interventions and successful resolutions of incidents can increase staff members' confidence.

- Use staff debriefings to identify areas requiring modification of administrative policy and procedures pertaining to the use of restraint or seclusion, and may serve to reduce use of restraint or seclusion (see Chapter 2).

- If there has been injury, meet with supervisory staff to evaluate the circumstances that caused the injury and develop a plan to prevent future injuries.

Documentation

Each incident of restraint or seclusion should be documented after the incident, and an incident report must be filed in the individual's permanent file. Documentation should include

- a description of what happened;
- date and time of day of occurrence;
- intervention used, reasons for use, and the duration of the intervention;
- children involved;
- caregivers or others involved, including full names, titles, and relationship to the child;
- witnesses to the incident;
- person making the report;
- any injury to the child including body chart or photo of any injuries;
- action taken by the provider;
- preventive actions to be taken in the future;
- any follow-up required; and
- documentation of supervisory or administrative review.

Follow-Up

Notification of the Individual's Family or Legal Guardian

The individual's family or legal guardian should be notified as soon as possible after a restraint or seclusion, or according to the wishes of the family.

Medical Treatment for Injuries Resulting from Restraint or Seclusion

When an injury results from restraint or seclusion, the following actions must be taken.

- Provide immediate medical treatment by qualified medical personnel to a child or youth who is injured during restraint or seclusion.

- Document these injuries in the individual's record.

- Provide immediate medical treatment by qualified medical personnel to staff who sustained injuries during the restraint or seclusion of a resident.

- Document these injuries in the child or youth's record and in the caregiver's record.

(See Chapter 4 for additional information concerning medical intervention and follow-up.)

Report of Death or Injury During or After Restraint or Seclusion

A provider should report to the appropriate law enforcement, regulatory, and accrediting agencies for investigation whenever a serious injury or death occurs during, or as a result of, a restrictive intervention. (See Chapter 2.)

Critical Incident Stress Debriefing

It is important to learn from, and process our experiences of working with, the people in our care. This is especially important when a situation has a high risk of harm to the person or, in fact, has harmed the person in our care. These situations are defined as critical incidents. Certain events are always considered traumatic to people and as such are called critical incidents. These events are physical or sexual assault, death or serious injury, witnessing abuse of a person in our care, natural disasters, building fires, riots, and hostage situations. People exposed to one or more critical incidents are subject to critical incident stress (Mitchell, 1983). While each person has a different threshold for critical incident stress, there are serious consequences from it. Bergmann and Queen (1987) describe it this way. Immediately after a critical incident, personnel may experience significant withdrawal from important people, activities, and job-related tasks. They may re-experience the event through flashbacks, suffer depression, have difficulty sleeping, and have nightmares. They may suffer anxiety, hyperalertness, and guilt, and may have difficulty returning to work. It is not uncommon for caregivers to say they have no feelings or feel dead inside or numb. Without appropriate action following a critical incident, severe and long-term consequences may result.

Critical incidents are emotionally traumatic to the people directly involved and, in some cases, to persons not directly involved.

Staff members should be provided with appropriate forums for discussion of the events and of their feelings. When necessary, counseling and follow-up should also be provided.

CHAPTER 4

Medical Issues

Introduction

When caregivers use seclusion and restraint techniques, they create additional potential for harm, including serious injury or death. The goal of caregivers must be, "First, do no harm." Restraint and seclusion, even when necessary, are high-risk interventions. The procedures are inherently dangerous and there are no absolutely safe techniques. However, there are ways to minimize the risks.

This chapter will provide, from a medical perspective, best practice guidelines on the use of restraint and seclusion. It will address the following areas:

- Nature and scope of restraint usage
- Medical or psychiatric risk assessments
- Monitoring restraint and seclusion
- Medical response to restraint-precipitated emergencies

Throughout this chapter, guidelines will be presented that are intended to be applicable to the use of restraint and seclusion in a wide range of settings—including psychiatric hospitals, residential treatment, group homes, boot camps, juvenile correction facilities, day treatment, educational programs, foster care, day care, and in-home services—most of which are not primarily medical facilities.

The Nature and Scope of Restraint Usage and Associated Injuries

Introduction and Scope

Restraint is a surprisingly widespread intervention in our society. While these guidelines focus on the use of restraint for behavioral safety for children and youth, it is important to understand that restraint techniques are used throughout the lifespan, ranging from the use of mechanical restraints in a neonatal intensive care unit to poseys in a hospice or a geriatric medical unit. While our focus is on behavioral health issues, restraints are also used in a medical and surgical context, and in the realms of policing, juvenile justice, corrections, and education.

An important distinction is often made between the uses of mechanical restraints for medical, as opposed to behavioral, purposes. While a philosophical distinction can be made, and there are usually physical differences in technique as well, there is still risk to the child.

Throughout these guidelines, it is stated explicitly that restraint should be used only to prevent severe harm or the risk of severe harm to a child or a child's potential victim. Restraint, however, continues to be used in some cases for different purposes, such as to impose discipline, punish, prevent property destruction, or inflict pain. Restraint is also sometimes applied as a result of inappropriate escalation between caregiver and child, and in police and correctional settings as a measure to prevent greater violence.

Restraint Usage

Restraints are used in the four different realms mentioned earlier: behavioral, medical/surgical, correctional/forensic, and educational. The remainder of this discussion will focus on the use of restraint during behavioral treatments and interventions, in any setting.

Patterns of use are known to vary from provider to provider and region to region. Intensive tracking of time of use and caregivers involved can reveal patterns of maximum use for individual children and units. Typical findings are that restraint use increases during unstructured time, such as weekends or evenings, or that some caregivers become overwhelmed and resort to the use of restraints before others do.

Within a setting, it is common to find that specific individuals are "high users" who are restrained much more than the average child. Some individuals in a setting may never be restrained, whereas others are restrained daily or even more frequently.

As the intensity of behavioral disturbance, especially violence, increases, so usually do the intensity, duration, and frequency of restraints. As these increase, the risk of child and caregiver injury and death also increases.

Injuries During Restraint

Injuries during restraint can occur to child or caregivers. These range in intensity from minor to severe or even fatal. It should not be assumed that if staff injuries significantly outweigh child injuries, restraint use in any given program is probably appropriate. There are no satisfactory norms for appropriate patterns of restraint use by child, age, or program type.

When the intensity and frequency of aggressive and violent behavior increases and the use of restraint increases, it is expected that the rate of injury will also increase. In any given setting, however, minor and minimal injuries should be predominate; severe, life-threatening, or fatal injuries should be nonexistent or rare.

Injuries can affect any system of the body, but those involving the brain, heart, or lungs are especially dangerous. No restraint system, hold, or use pattern is safe for all children at all times. All, even properly applied, can be fatal. The reason is that, negligent practice aside, injuries and fatalities occur because of the interaction between the restraint hold or technique used, the intensity and duration of restraint, the medical condition of the child, and the attentiveness and procedural technique of the restraining caregiver. In general, most or all of these factors have to go awry to cause a life-threatening or fatal outcome. The combination of factors dangerous for one child's restraint, however, could be optimal for another child. Simple banning of "forbidden" techniques is not expected to end severe or fatal restraint-associated injuries.

Some types of injury are known to be particularly prominent during restraint. In younger children, especially, there is vulnerability to joint dislocation and long bone fractures. Techniques exerting pressure on the limbs can cause peripheral nerve injuries. Certain holds can intensify trauma in previously abused individuals.

Restraint-associated asphyxia, also known as positional asphyxia, is particularly dangerous because it is a major cause of restraint-associated death. Asphyxia occurs when lack of air intake deprives the child of oxygen. Lack of oxygen, in turn, eventually triggers a cardiac arrest followed by brain death. Prevention is usually as simple as making sure that the restrained child can, or is allowed to, breathe. This requires that caregivers be well trained, that the child's medical risk factors have been correctly assessed, and that monitoring during the restraint is appropriate.

Beyond the generalities listed above, there are a host of special conditions that can predispose a child to a dangerous outcome. Examples include hemophilia, which increases the risk of bleeding; asthma, which increases the risk of insufficient oxygenation; and hepatitis, which increases the risk of abdominal injury.

Prescribed and over-the-counter medications and substances may increase the risk of negative outcome. Acute substance-induced intoxication and vomiting are particularly associated with restraint-associated asphyxia. Medications for the treatment of asthma can create a predisposition toward vomiting or cardiac arrhythmia.

Psychiatric medications and anticonvulsants are often sedative and can increase the risk of asphyxia.

Anything that compresses or restricts the chest or stomach also increases the risk of asphyxia. Common examples include simple obesity and certain types of physical holds.

Restraints for the sole purpose of causing pain are ethically indefensible. Techniques should be applied in a way that does not intentionally cause pain. (See Chapter 1 and 3 for information about prohibited practices.)

Maximizing and Minimizing Risk

Because no restraint is completely safe, a best practices approach to restraint is likely to minimize injuries. Once it is accepted that any restraint can cause injury and death and that dangerous outcomes are due to multiple predisposing factors, combined with multiple safety system failures, it becomes clear that the task of increasing restraint safety is one of minimizing risk factors and maximizing safety factors. For any given provider this will require developing its own best practices or adopting best practices developed elsewhere.

Factors that Increase Risk of Restraint-Associated Injuries

Since severe injury and death are rare outcomes during restraint, any restraint should be approached with the intent of reducing even further the likelihood of those outcomes. By planning for each child and generating an individualized restraint plan on admission (see Chapter 3) that takes into account his or her personal risk factors, the provider should be able to achieve that goal.

The following factors increase the risk of poor outcome during restraint:

- Smaller size
- Larger size
- Younger age
- Obesity
- Previous emotional trauma
- Child-specific medical or surgical conditions
- Pregnancy
- Increased intensity of restraint
- Increased duration of restraint
- Increased frequency of restraint
- Psychiatric medications
- Cardiac medications
- Asthma medications
- Dehydration
- Overheating
- Overexercising
- Chest compression or restriction
- Abdominal compression or restriction

- Neck compression or restriction

- Asthma

- Respiratory disease

- Other chest disease

- Kypho-scoliosis

- Other neck or spine disease

- Sedation

- Sedative medications

- Vomiting

- Full stomach

- Acute intoxication due to substances

- Agitation, exercise, oxygen deficit (demonstrated by increased respiratory rate) just prior to restraint

- Agitation in restraint

- Inadequate facial monitoring during restraint

- Refusing to heed child's complaint of "I can't breathe," or "You're hurting me" during restraint—even if it is false and manipulative

The risk factors above may apply to any of the following restraint techniques:

- Standing restraint

- Prone restraint

- Supine restraint

- Basket holds

- Physical escorts

High-Risk Clusters

Some combinations of restraint risk factors appear to be particularly high risk. Several of these high-risk clusters are given below.

Respiratory	agitation; asthma; abdominal or chest compression/restriction; sedative medications; complaint of difficulty breathing
Cardiac	agitation; stimulant medication; cardiac disease
Trauma	prone restraint; restraining caregiver is the same gender as a previous abuser; prolonged caregiver-child physical contact
Abdominal	agitation; hepatitis; abdominal compression; bleeding disorder

These few examples make the point that restraints are most safe when individualized for each child, and most unsafe when they are not.

Safety Factors that Decrease Restraint-Associated Injuries

The following list includes factors that decrease the risk of injury to a child during restraint. In some jurisdictions, some of these are mandatory. All of them should be useful in reducing the risk of injury and death.

- Provide adequate caregiver ratios
- Provide adequate staff training
- Optimize asthma/respiratory status as soon as possible after admission
- Minimize sedation as soon as possible after admission
- Plan for child-specific medical or surgical conditions
- Develop individualized restraint plans
- Avoid power struggles
- Restrain only for safety
- Decrease the intensity of restraint
- Decrease the duration of restraint
- Decrease the frequency of restraint
- Monitor respiration and skin color
- Maintain hydration
- Prevent overheating

- Restrain child positioned in a chair
- Uncover the face
- Monitor the child's face during the restraint
- Heed any complaint of "I can't breathe" during restraint—even if it is false and manipulative—and break the restraint

The realization that no restraint or method of applying restraints is always safe for all children is very daunting for caregivers. For those nevertheless required to apply restraints, the goal becomes one of minimizing risk rather than simply doing things "the right way." A best practice analysis teaches us that to minimize risk we should avoid unnecessary restraints; minimize restraint frequency, duration, and intensity; avoid certain dangerous practices that have no unique clinical utility; minimize known risk factors; and maximize known safety factors.

Medical or Psychiatric Assessments

Numerous medical and psychiatric conditions can pose a danger for a child or youth if he or she were to be physically restrained. If any medical or psychiatric conditions are discovered during the assessment process that could pose a danger to the child, it is strongly recommended that the individual be reassessed by the proper licensed practitioner prior to restraint application. Each child must be completely assessed before application of any form of restraint to determine that no apparent danger to the child exists. The list of potential medical and psychiatric conditions that could prove to be a danger to a child or youth being restrained is lengthy and impossible to include in its entirety. The list in this section is intended to alert the caregiver to the possibility of a negative outcome if no further assessment is obtained before applying a restraint.

A physical assessment and examination by a proper licensed practitioner should be performed before, or at the time of, the child's admission. This assessment should determine whether any preexisting medical illnesses or conditions exist that would prohibit or limit the use of certain restraint techniques. It is further recommended that each provider develop a form to be signed by a licensed practitioner that requires review of restraint and seclusion practices for that child.

When an assessment identifies medical illnesses and conditions that indicate risk, the results should be communicated to all staff members. The child's individual restraint plan must identify prescriptive interventions that minimize risk and any interventions that are prohibited for that child.

Medical Illnesses and Conditions that Affect an Individual's Response to Seclusion and Restraint

Respiratory illnesses and conditions such as asthma, obesity, and pregnancy are medical illnesses and conditions that distort restraint responses and increase risks. Conditions that would place a child in danger if restrained include, but are not limited to, the following:

Cardiac

- **Myocarditis**—inflammation of the middle layer of the heart that is associated with certain infections. Heavy physical activity could cause an increase in oxygen demand, which would cause a rapid heart rate. This could lead to dangerous heart rhythms.

- **Heart murmurs**—soft blowing or rasping sounds heard when listening to the heart sounds. Heart murmurs can be pathologic and dangerous if not identified properly.

- **Myocardial infarction**—a heart attack. Although this condition may be rare in children, excess physical activity could lead to cardiac arrest and death.

- **Angina pectoris**—a severe pain in the chest and a sensation of constriction around the heart. This is usually caused by a deficiency of oxygen to the heart muscle that will lead to dangerous heart rhythms.

- **Marfan's syndrome**—a hereditary condition in which the aorta is weak and prone to the formation of an aneurysm. During physical activity, the aneurysm could rupture and cause death.

- **Pacemaker**—an artificial electrical stimulation of the heart muscle to expand and contract. Physical activity could cause one of the leads to be disconnected from the ventricle, which would lead to dangerous heart rhythms and possibly death.

- **Anticoagulant therapy**—the use of blood thinners. Bruising during physical activity could cause excessive bleeding.

- **Hypertension**—high blood pressure. High blood pressure during physical activity could cause a stroke.

- **Gunshot or stab wounds of the chest**—any penetrating wound to the chest may leave scar tissue or a foreign object in the chest or heart that could prove fatal if physical restraint is attempted.

Pulmonary

- **Bronchial asthma**—a constriction of the bronchial airway. Severe asthma will cause difficulty breathing and could lead to respiratory distress should an attack occur during physical activity.

- **Temporary tracheotomy**—a surgical incision into the trachea due to obstruction of the airway. Physical activity could dislodge the tracheal tube and cause respiratory arrest and death.

- **Fractured ribs**—a rib fracture poses the danger of puncturing a lung, causing it to collapse.

- **Obstructive pulmonary disease**—a disease process that causes shortness of breath and difficulty breathing. Physical restraints involving the chest could cause extreme difficulty breathing and lead to respiratory or cardiac arrest and death.

Musculoskeletal

- **Fractures**—recent or healing fractures can pose a significant risk to the individual. Orthopedic hardware (screws, nails, plates) can become dislodged during the restraint process, causing more severe injury. Harrington rods (used for correction of scoliosis) pose a danger; if these rods are bent, significant secondary health issues will result for the individual.

- **Osteogenesis imperfecta**—an inherited condition that results in less bone density, thereby making it easier for bones to break. Fractures can result from physical restraint procedures.

- **Scoliosis**—an abnormal curvature of the spine. This disease process poses a severe danger to the individual. Physical restraint procedures can result in further damage to the spine itself, or cause significant neurological problems.

- **Kyphosis (hunchback)**—an abnormal curvature of the spine. Physical restraint procedures could lead to excessive pain, fracture, and possible neurological damage.

- **Osteomyelitis**—inflammation of the bone marrow. The danger with this disease is that muscles are usually rigid. Physical restraint may cause muscle tearing, bleeding, and spread of the infection to the entire system.

Gastrointestinal

- **Hiatal hernia**—protrusion of the stomach into the chest cavity through the diaphragm. This condition could lead to respiratory compromise during the physical restraint procedure.

- **Ostomies** (colostomies, iliostomies, ureterostomies, etc.)—the formation of an artificial stoma for elimination. Human waste products may be spilled during the restraint process, or the surgical process may be damaged, causing bleeding and infections.

- **Gastroesophageal reflux**—reflux of stomach contents into the esophagus. Vomiting may result from a physical restraint, and the individual could aspirate the vomitus into the lungs.

- **Abdominal surgery**—recent surgery to the abdomen poses many dangers to the individual. There may be a dehiscence (opening) of the surgical wound, excessive bleeding, infection, and a reversal of the surgical repair.

Endocrine

- **Diabetes mellitus**—inadequate production of insulin. This poses severe risks for the individual. A noncompliant diabetic who does not take his or her insulin may go into ketoacidosis, which could be a life-threatening consequence.

Neurologic

- **Epilepsy or other seizure disorder**—a disorder of cerebral function that is characterized by convulsive seizures. Seizures may result from high stimulus (physical or mechanical restraint procedures). Airways can be compromised; vomiting may result.

Psychiatric

- **Posttraumatic stress disorder**—the development of characteristic symptoms after a psychologically traumatic event. Approaching an individual with PTSD may trigger a recurrence of the event and lead to the exhibition of aggressive behavior.

- **Abuse**—victims of physical, emotional, sexual, and psychological abuse are at a high risk during physical restraint. The trauma of restraint could do further harm to these individuals.

- **Neuroleptic malignant syndrome (NMS)**—a potentially fatal idiosyncratic complication of neuroleptic treatment. The frequency of NMS is rare, but the outcome can be disastrous. Clinical signs of this syndrome include a high fever (102 to 104 degrees), rapid heart rate, difficulty breathing, profuse sweating, rigidity, an altered state of consciousness, and either a rise or lowering of blood pressure. Health care employees need to understand that anyone being treated with neuroleptic therapy is susceptible to developing this syndrome, which can be fatal. It would be best practice to monitor any person taking neuroleptic medication for signs of this rare, but deadly syndrome.

Obstetrical

- **Pregnancy**—pregnancy poses severe danger to the individual in a restraint situation. Takedowns can cause spontaneous abortion, tearing of the placenta, which would lead to severe bleeding and possibly death for both the mother and fetus, as well as possible birth defects to the fetus. Pregnant young women may also develop toxemia, which would be life threatening to the mother and baby. A pregnant young woman must be evaluated by an obstetrician before any restraint procedure.

  Prone (face down) restraint for young women in their second and third trimesters of pregnancy should be prohibited in order to avoid undue pressure on the developing fetus. Any standing techniques that do not allow the restrained individual to maintain balance should be avoided, as a fall would place both the individual and the fetus at risk of injury.

Congenital Problems

- **Down's syndrome**—the presence of an extra chromosome, which causes mental retardation. This syndrome poses a significant danger to the individual during a restraint procedure because there is high danger of dislocation of the first cervical vertebra (Atlantoaxial instability), which would cause respiration to cease.

Pharmacological Issues

- It would be impossible to list all of the individual and combinations of medications that could cause drowsiness, lethargy, impaired respiration, and impaired function. All medication regimens should be assessed by the proper licensed practitioner before placing any individual into a restraint.

Substance Abuse

- Any individual with a history of drug or alcohol abuse must be considered a high risk to restrain. Individuals may exhibit symptoms of withdrawal, which would place them in danger of physical harm while being restrained. Vomiting, hyperventilation, seizures, and involuntary muscle movement are but a few of the symptoms that could place the individual in jeopardy during a restraint process.

Assessment is the key to best practice when that practice involves restraint. Individuals must be assessed continuously for any conditions that would place them in imminent danger while being restrained. Therefore, policies and procedures need to reflect a thorough assessment process before applying any form of restraint.

An individual who becomes agitated during physical or mechanical restraint or seclusion is under a great deal of physical stress and may exhibit signs of that distress. In order to minimize risk and harm to individuals, provider-should train all caregivers to use specific monitoring procedures that assess for any sign of distress. Table 1 was developed to assist providers in developing policies and procedures. It reviews, by bodily system, the signs of distress.

Table 1: Restraint Responses that Indicate Distress

System	Signs of Distress
Circulatory	Extremities are cold to the touch Blue tinge to nail beds Blue tinge to the area around the mouth Flushed or ashen face
Respiratory	Rapid, shallow breathing Panting Grunting Blue tinge to nail beds Blue tinge to the area around the mouth Nasal flaring Absence of breathing
Neurological	Confusion/disorientation Seizure Vomiting Difficulty breathing Unconsciousness Unequal pupil size Headaches
Gastrointestinal	Vomiting Constipation Diarrhea
Musculoskeletal	Joint swelling Pain Redness Bruising

Table 2 reviews risks and concerns by restraint position. Providers should review this table to further enhance education of caregivers about monitoring techniques. Special consideration should be given to the size and weight of the individual(s) restraining, in relation to the size and weight of the individual being restrained—based on the risk and concerns outlined in Table 2.

Table 2: Positional Risk

POSITION	RISK CONCERN
Standing	Breathing may be restricted Possibility of bruises, strained muscles, or other musculoskeletal injuries Person(s) initiating the restraint may exert too much pressure or be too forceful
Sitting	Breathing may be restricted Cardiac and/or respiratory arrest Possibility of neck and back injuries Possibility of abrasions, bruises, strained muscles, or other musculoskeletal injuries Person(s) initiating the restraint may exert too much pressure or be too forceful, particularly over the neck or spine If chair is used, chair may overturn
Prone (face down)	Possibility of abrasions, bruises, or other musculoskeletal injuries, particularly to the face Possibility of neck and back injuries Difficulty breathing, including respiratory arrest Cardiac arrest Decreased circulation to lower extremities Surface of floor may not be padded Person(s) initiating the restraint may exert too much pressure or be too forceful, particularly over the chest and neck, or may place too much weight on a limb or joint Person being restrained may bang head or struggle against hold Note: obese individuals are more susceptible to these risks
Supine (Face-up)	Possibility of abrasions, bruises, strained muscles, or other musculoskeletal injuries Difficulty breathing including respiratory arrest
Supine (Face-up)	Possibility of asphyxiation if individual vomits Possibility of biting self Surface of floor may not be padded Person(s) initiating the restraint may exert too much pressure or be too forceful, particularly over the chest and neck, or may place too much weight on a limb or joint Person being restrained may struggle against hold

Monitoring, Assessment, and Maintenance of Physical Integrity During Restraint and Seclusion

The task force recommends that certain assessments and monitoring activities be used during any behavior management technique. These assessments and monitoring activities can be performed by any members of the agency's staff, provided they have received appropriate training and are periodically evaluated for demonstrated competence in these duties. This face-to-face assessment and monitoring should address the child's health status and bodily integrity, as well as his or her physical and emotional needs.

Consciousness, respiration, agitation, mental status, skin color, and skin integrity should be monitored continuously while the child or youth is in restraint or seclusion.

Table 3 lists recommended guidelines for assessments and monitoring that need to be done in addition to the continuous monitoring. Each assessment or monitoring activity is listed by type of intervention, appropriateness for use, and recommended frequency. Providers should always consult their own medical advisors for any other suggested additions to the table. Individual restraint plans may call for more frequent monitoring, based on an individual's medical condition(s). Providers should also consider limitations to restraint procedures based on their ability to provide the necessary monitoring, as specified.

Special monitors related to medical illnesses and conditions should include fetal monitoring for pregnant females.

Minimal Requirements For Comfort and Physical Integrity

There are unique concerns regarding the rights of individuals during behavior management techniques. These rights, and a general concern for the well-being of children and youth in restraint or seclusion call upon us to ensure that certain needs are met on a regular basis during these procedures. Caregivers assigned to monitor children and youth should be aware of these

Table 3: Monitoring Guidelines by Procedure Type

Type of Monitor	Type of Intervention				
	Chemical	**Mechanical**	**Seclusion**	**Physical**	**Time-out**
Temperature	Every 2 hours	Every 2 hours			
Pulse	Every 15 min.	Every 15 min.	Every 15 min.	Every 15 min.	
Respiration	Every 15 min.	Every 15 min.	Every 15 min.	Every 15 min.	Every 15 min.
Blood Pressure	Every 2 hours	Every 2 hours	Every 2 hours (if level of agitation allows)	Every 2 hours	
Level of Consciousness	Every 15 min.	Every 15 min.	Every 15 min.	Every 15 min.	Every 15 min.
Level of Agitation	Every 15 min.	Every 15 min.	Every 15 min.	Every 15 min.	Every 15 min.
Mental Status	Every 15 min.	Every 15 min.	Every 15 min.	Every 15 min.	Every 15 min.
Skin Color		Every 15 min.		Every 15 min.	
Skin Integrity		Every 15 min.		Every 15 min.	
Temperature of Extremities		Every 15 min.		Every 15 min.	
Swelling of Extremities		Every 15 min.		Every 15 min.	
Movement of Extremities		Every 15 min.		Every 15 min.	

rights and should provide for these needs to be met with the following minimum frequencies:

Hydration	Every 2 hours
Nutrition	At established mealtimes
Elimination	Every 2 hours
Range of Motion	Every 2 hours

An individual's restraint plan may require more frequent intervals, depending upon the child's medical history, condition, and medications.

Emergency Response to Restraint-Precipitated Emergencies

Even the most professional behavioral management interventions can sometimes lead to accidents for which emergency medical assistance is required. Providers must establish emergency response protocols to be used in conjunction with behavior management interventions.

Protocols should include the following areas.

Internal Response

- Because behavioral management incidents are often unpredictable and many times very short in duration, medical personnel may not be immediately available. Thus, caregivers should be certified in First Aid and CPR and trained in health issues related to the use of restraint and seclusion. They should also be knowledgeable about any medical conditions unique to individuals in their care that prohibit the use of physical intervention.

- Incidents that include the use of behavior interventions that physically restrict the individual should prompt communication with available internal medical resources for support as necessary.

- When possible, available internal medical personnel should monitor incidents in which physically restrictive interventions are employed.

- Staff members identified as medical resources should have the authority to continue or stop a specific intervention based on health issues.

- Internal medical personnel should examine individuals as soon as possible after the incident has ended, when such examination is deemed necessary.

- The follow-up medical assessment should prompt outside medical assessment and treatment, as necessary.

- Universal precautions should be employed.

External Response

- In advance of a medical emergency, external medical personnel should be identified, and emergency assistance procedures with these resources should be established. Procedures should include communication, transportation, agency access, back-up in case the identified personnel are unavailable, and follow-up review.

- Medical records, parental permission, and insurance information must be available for use by external resources. Providers are advised to create medical summaries that include the above information for all individuals. All staff should know how to access this information when needed.

- Judgment about requesting external assistance should rest with the staff involved in the incident and/or the identified internal medical resource. Requests for external assistance should be based on their assessment of the individual's current health status.

- Emergency response protocol should also include procedures to guarantee communication with the individual's parent or guardian and with licensing authority, as required by statute or regulation. (See Chapters 1 and 2.)

- A provider representative should accompany individuals who are transported to an external emergency resource.

Follow-Up

- Emergency response protocols should include requirements to communicate with staff regarding the emergency. Initially, such communication should be general information, to respect confidentiality issues as well as protect the integrity of the investigation.

- Communication with the public (press, news media) should follow established procedure. One person should be identified as the provider's spokesperson.

CHAPTER 5

Professional Development and Support for Staff & Caregivers

Introduction

Every day, children with increasingly complex and severe problems enter child-serving systems. Because working with children is, by nature, a labor-intensive field, our systems of care can expand to meet these needs only to the extent that providers are able to recruit, train, and retain additional numbers of highly trained and motivated staff. Dealing successfully with children who exhibit a wide range of behavioral problems requires an educated, experienced, and committed professional workforce. This must remain the goal of all child-serving agencies, public and private alike.

Mission and Vision

Competent and motivated staff members are the key to effective work with children and youth. Developing a skilled and enthusiastic workforce must be the central purpose of every provider's professional development and support program. To meet this goal, providers must create workplace environments that embody the following three critical themes.

1. Caregivers must be connected and powerfully committed to the unifying mission of the organization. The mission of work with children is a compelling one that can capture the hearts and minds of staff. To make the mission a reality, agencies must clearly communicate it to all personnel, link it directly to the work that staff members do on a day-to-day basis, ensure that policies and procedures conform to the mission, and celebrate performance that exemplifies the mission.

2. The provider must place strong emphasis on learning, innovation, and development at both the individual and organizational levels. Providers that promote ongoing professional and lifelong learning opportunities will produce more skilled workers who are committed to

the provider and the field, innovative in their approach, and who produce more effective outcomes for children and families.

3. The provider must emphasize relationships, partnerships, and teamwork to carry out the mission, vision, and values of the organization. To be effective, caregivers and providers must be skilled in and committed to working as teammates and partners. These skills are essential for effective work with children and families, coworkers, other service providers, and contracting and regulatory agencies.

Professional development within this context includes at least four major components:

- recruitment and hiring,
- orientation and preservice training,
- in-service training, and
- resources and other supports.

The sections that follow discuss the critical contributions made by each of these areas.

Recruitment and Hiring

Recruitment

The primary goal of recruitment is to find qualified individuals who share a common value system with the agency. To accomplish this goal, providers should recruit potential staff using a wide variety of methods, including newspapers, the Internet, colleges, and current staff referrals. In addition, all recruitment efforts should include clear statements of the provider's mission and values, as well as the specific duties of the positions advertised, and the required qualifications. This not only serves as the initial step in educating potential employees, but also serves to educate the public to the provider's philosophic beliefs and values.

First impressions are significant. During the initial contact with potential employees, employers should explain enthusiastically the provider's purpose and services, and should provide a clear and balanced description of the realities of the position being offered. The provider should also describe briefly the nature of the workplace environment as well as opportunities for advancement within the organization. By presenting this information at the beginning of the hiring process, employers give potential employees the information they need to decide whether their values, expertise, interests, and long-term goals correspond with the needs, philosophy, and practices of the agency. The initial contact is also an opportunity for the provider to ask questions to help ascertain whether this candidate possesses the requisite qualifications and shares the values and beliefs of the agency.

Interviewing

To conduct an effective interview, a provider must first have a clear idea of the kinds of people it wishes to employ. That is, it must clearly identify the experience, skills, attitudes, and values that are most highly related to successful job performance. Then, a significant portion of the interview should be structured to assess directly the extent to which the candidate possesses those qualities. Such an interview process requires the development of open-ended questions that are designed to ascertain the compatibility of the candidate's beliefs, values, and experience with the provider's mission, practices, procedures, policies, and philosophies, including those related to behavior guidance. These questions should be asked of all candidates, and candidates' answers should be rated in a structured, systematic manner.

A second goal of the interview process is to ensure that the potential candidate is familiar with the specific duties of the particular position being sought, as well as with other critical aspects of the agency. The interviewer should include discussion of the children served by the provider, the types of behaviors they may exhibit, and the range of interventions used. This portion of the interview is accomplished best through a combination of discussion and written materials. Special attention should be focused on how the agency mission and values relate directly to the day-to-day expectations of employees. This discussion can be enhanced by the use of program tours, videos of workers engaged in performing typical job duties, and review of written job descriptions. Also helpful at this point is a discussion of the agency's career ladder and available training and educational opportunities. Such detailed information will help candidates understand the job for which they are applying, their potential for advancement within the agency, and the degree of match between their skills and abilities and the provider's needs.

Orientation and Preservice Training

Foundation

Caregivers who are most involved in the direct supervision of children will require comprehensive training on the continuum of interventions that may be necessary to manage behaviors. Necessary elements of this training are covered in the section below.

All personnel should be aware of the philosophy, rules, policies and procedures, intervention modalities used, and the provider's expectations for everyone who is working with children. This information should be conveyed through agency training initiatives that begin with orientation and preservice training. It should lay a foundation for further training in specific job-related duties and responsibilities.

When given a common framework for understanding the provider's approaches to managing client behaviors, all staff members will help create an environment of respect, consistency, and support for one another, as well as for the children and young people served by the agency.

Content

All personnel hired by the agency should complete orientation training that includes:

- overall agency treatment philosophy and approach;
- agency philosophy of behavior management;
- basic information about behaviors children may exhibit;
- identification of early warning signs that indicate children may become disruptive or aggressive and how these observations are to be reported;

- importance of professionalism in dealing with children, families, and others;
- interventions employed by caregivers to prevent, deescalate, safely manage, and follow up children's behaviors;
- roles and expectations of various personnel in preventing and responding to crisis situations;
- documentation requirements;
- working as part of a team;
- provider policies and procedures relating to crisis prevention or intervention and response to client behaviors; and
- emergency response procedures.

Staff Training Plans

During orientation, each employee should be made aware of the plan for his or her particular ongoing training and professional development. Plans should be developed between the employee and supervisor, and should be based on their roles and responsibilities in the program.

For caregivers and supervisors, ongoing training should require in-depth training in each of the elements covered in orientation training.

Other staff members whose involvement with clients is not as "direct" (i.e. support staff, medical, clinical, etc.) may not require the same level of training in these areas. They should, however, be made aware of the intervention framework established in training so they can understand and support the procedures and interventions being utilized by caregivers, particularly those elements that impact their own areas of responsibility.

By identifying the plan for ongoing training, staff members will be assured that they will have resources to obtain information and build the skills necessary to carry out their responsibilities. This is critical in recruitment and retention efforts, in creating a positive work environment, and increasing staff confidence and professionalism.

In-Service Training

Formal training programs, typically delivered in classroom or workshop style settings, are a necessary, though not sufficient, component of overall professional development. Without adequate training, workers will generally not be able to perform the many complex and difficult duties required of them. But training programs alone are not enough. They must be implemented in the context of an overall effort that devotes the personnel and fiscal resources necessary to ensure significant supervision and support.

Within this context, the ultimate goal of professional development is for staff members to perform more effectively in their actual work settings. Top quality formal training programs can play a significant role in this effort. They do this by targeting three critical goals:

- Providing personnel with the information necessary to perform their jobs well;

- Ensuring that workers' attitudes and values about children and their work are consistent with the provider's views;

- Teaching staff the specific skills and competencies they will need to perform at a high level.

Formal training will only be effective to the extent that it attends to the six principles of adult learning listed below.

- Training should be developed from an assessment of individuals' training needs, preferably one that involves workers in the process. Providers must determine the most critical staff competencies, assess current worker capabilities in those areas, and target the most pressing competencies for training.

- Adult participants should be treated as resources. Adult learners bring a wealth of knowledge and experience to training activities. Quality training will ensure that worker abilities are used throughout the sessions.

- Overall training effectiveness is greatly increased when participants actively use and practice the knowledge and skills they are learning during the sessions.

- Training should occur in a comfortable learning environment. Adult learners need to feel physically and emotionally comfortable in order for serious learning to take place.

- Effective instruction will systematically incorporate teaching strategies that target a range of learning styles appropriate for adult learners.

- Trainers should always remember that time is a valuable commodity and cannot be squandered. Training should target directly relevant skills, start and end on time, and be briskly paced.

Model for Training Delivery

A comprehensive model for training delivery must address the following question: "Who will deliver how much of what, when, where, and how?"

Who?

Good trainers are hard to find. This is because they must possess at least four critical sets of skills:

- They must be experts (or at least be highly knowledgeable) in the specific content area being taught. They must have both a conceptual grasp of the information and the ability to apply it to real situations.

- They must know how the content they are teaching relates to other program components and fits into the overall services being provided. Otherwise, they will not be able to help workers determine how and when particular skills should be applied.

- Good trainers should have significant actual experience in applying the knowledge and skills being taught in work settings. This will enable them to provide multiple examples to illustrate how and when the skills can be best applied.

- Trainers must be skilled group facilitators. They must be comfortable and competent in front of an audience, knowledgeable about adult learning principles, and capable of dealing with the wide range of issues and problems that can arise during training sessions.

New trainers will need to be taught these skills.

Although finding good trainers is critical, it is also important to expose workers to a variety of trainers. A comprehensive training program should include trainers from all levels of the organization, including peers, supervisors, and other agency experts, as well as external experts from other organizations and colleges. In addition, the use of cotrainers can greatly enhance training effectiveness, especially for less-experienced trainers.

How Much?

The amount of training provided must obviously depend on the need and on the topics being taught. There is no magic formula. Clearly, training for workers must meet licensing requirements for specific topics, as well as for yearly totals. However, given that caregivers often lack relevant preservice training and experience, it is clear that they may need much more training than what is required for licensing. It is ironic that the most skilled and credentialed professionals in our agencies often get the most training, while training for direct care workers often barely meets the licensing minimums.

Almost as important as the amount of training is the need for it to be systematic and ongoing. Agencies should develop comprehensive training plans for all levels of workers and make sure that training is available on a consistent basis over time. Providers should establish annual training requirements for each position, in compliance with regulatory requirements and accreditation standards. Because it seems more efficient, there is a tendency for training to be done in large segments that are widely spaced. There is considerable evidence that briefer, more frequent training sessions are more effective in producing improved worker performance on the job.

What?

The roles of agency direct service workers cover an extremely broad range of responsibilities. As such, targeting the knowledge and skills that such workers must possess is not an easy task. The first step in designing a comprehensive training program is to conduct a needs assessment—one that includes licensing requirements, as well as analysis of both basic and advanced critical worker competencies. Once these competencies have been identified, then detailed curricula can be developed for each competency. These curricula should include specific goals, methods, activities, and evaluation procedures.

Caregivers need a broad range of information and skills to work well with children who have emotional and behavioral problems. The list below summarizes some of the knowledge and skills needed to successfully prevent, minimize, and manage behavioral incidents.

Knowledge of:

- Agency mission and treatment philosophy
- Children and families served, including special needs
- Sensitivity to cultural differences
- Basic roles and responsibilities of caregivers
- Relevant provider policies and procedures
- Systems and laws governing the field

Skills in:

- Relationship building
- Listening and communication
- Developing and implementing activity programs
- Designing and implementing routines
- Managing transitions
- Managing personal boundaries
- Understanding and analyzing problem behavior
- Teaching social and anger management skills
- Implementing provider behavior management systems
- Setting clear expectations
- Praising and reinforcing children
- Early detection of conflict situations
- Interventions to minimize potential conflicts
- Conflict resolution
- Implementing physical escorts
- Implementing actual physical restraints
- Monitoring children's health status during restraints

- Using seclusion procedures
- Debriefing following a critical incident
- First aid and emergency medical procedures
- Administering and documenting medication
- Documenting interventions and incidents

When?

Effective providers place great emphasis on continuous learning. Training should be ongoing throughout every individual's employment. Training should begin as soon as the orientation is completed. Some providers tend to overwhelm new workers with too much training too early in their employment. Lacking sufficient work experience, workers often fail to understand the context and need for the skills they are being taught, which seriously compromises their ability to master many important skills.

The most effective training programs consist of frequent, brief training offerings that are repeated as needed to ensure that staff members are mastering the critical skills.

More advanced training programs for experienced workers are also important. This ensures that workers do not simply repeat material they have already mastered; it also challenges them to improve their skills even further.

Where?

Many organizations lack good facilities and other resources for training. Therefore, much provider training is conducted in cramped settings that lack sufficient workspace and materials. The inadvertent communication to workers is that training is not worth the investment, a message providers must struggle not to send, as it greatly reduces the effectiveness of training efforts.

Providers should work hard to locate good space for training, renovate areas to make them more conducive to learning, and provide trainers with the materials and equipment needed to maximize the learning experience. If adequate space is not available at a provider site, it is often possible to locate free or inexpensive training facilities outside (e.g., other agencies, schools, libraries, and community centers). These external sites also have the advantage of isolating trainees from day-to-day work demands, which increases their ability to focus attention on the topics at hand.

How?

Adult learning principles suggest that training programs should include a wide range of teaching methodologies to maximize learning for all the participants. The ideal training format includes the following:

- some lecture to provide information;
- significant discussion and activities designed to enable trainees to better integrate the material into their repertoires;
- demonstration of behavior management interventions;
- modeling of new skills;
- participant role-playing, including practice of behavior management interventions;
- discussion and feedback to trainees regarding their performance of new skills;
- action planning, where trainees identify specific skills they want to transfer to their work sites, as well as strategies for doing so successfully; and
- evaluation of the relevance and effectiveness of the training process.

There is a powerful tendency for lecture formats to dominate training. Providers must work diligently to ensure that their training curricula provide trainers with numerous alternative-teaching methodologies.

Supplemental Training Programs

Even a well-designed agency training plan will fail to meet all the training needs of some groups of staff and some individuals. For this reason, it is recommended that providers also devise structures to supplement the overall training plan with additional programs, designed to meet those needs. These supplemental training options can be identified in a number of ways: at the request of involved staff, as a result of quality improvement measures, or at the recommendation of a supervisor or program manager. Supplemental training could consist of slight modifications of previous trainings, more advanced training in a previously addressed area, or an entire new curriculum in an area not previously trained. In addition to supplemental training, staff may require additional resources to better meet children's needs. Such resources could include additional written information, program materials or equipment, and consultation regarding specific issues or problems.

Professionalization and Certification

One of the factors contributing to the workforce crisis in children's services is the lack of professionalization and opportunities for advancement in the field of child care. Significant attention to training within agencies, building training completion into provider career ladders, and development of provider-based certification will help alleviate this problem. However, when training does not lead to a certification or credential that is recognized across agency boundaries, the ultimate effect on the field is likely to be minimal.

There are several local and regional certification programs being discussed across the United States, and the Association of Child and Youth Care Professionals is working on a national certification model. These efforts should be encouraged, and providers should be working now to develop training programs that will meet or approximate the guidelines established by these organizations.

Resources and Support

Supervision

Although careful hiring, quality orientation, and in-service training programs are essential in ensuring that staff have been introduced to the skills they need to perform their jobs, there is no guarantee that staff members have mastered the skills or that they will use them consistently on a day-to-day basis. Ensuring skill mastery and consistent use are typically the responsibility of the supervisors, who provide day-to-day on the job training and support for caregivers. For supervisors to ensure that caregivers are performing effectively, the following conditions must apply:

- Supervisors must complete all agency training sessions attended by the caregivers they supervise in order to ensure an understanding of the philosophy and intervention strategies taught.

- In addition to being highly skilled workers, supervisors must be trained comprehensively to perform their supervisory functions. This includes, at a minimum, training in such topics as coaching, providing feedback, team building, staff support, disciplinary actions, leadership, meeting management, and conflict resolution.

- Supervisors must receive consistent supervision and support themselves, in both individual and group settings.

- Supervisors should be charged with putting systems in place to ensure that the concepts taught in training can be effectively, efficiently, and realistically applied in the workplace.

- Trainers should provide to supervisors a listing of ongoing training opportunities and course objectives.

- Supervisors should receive documentation when supervisees attend training. Documentation should include, but not be limited to, copies of each employee's attendance record and any completed testing and evaluation utilized in training. Trainers should also provide to supervisors recommendations for further training and skill development of employees.

Individual Staff Development Plans and Accountability

An annual plan, based on job responsibilities, should be established with each employee to identify ongoing training needs. Ongoing training needs should include the provider's training courses as well as independent skill development through review of written resources, practice, mentoring by other staff, attendance at conferences, or other methods. The expectations held by the agency, including how caregivers interact with clients and intervene in disruptive situations, should be clearly identified and supported by agency policies and procedures.

Staff members should be encouraged to communicate whether the training and resources provided are helping them to perform according to expectations. When employees identify additional training needs, supervisors should consult with the provider staff responsible for training, to determine where other resources are available to meet these needs. The additional training or resources identified should be consistent with the provider's training framework, so as to be cohesive with all previous training and the training of other staff.

APPENDIX A

Best Practice Task Force

Kathy Barbell, Director
Resource Family Center
The Casey Family Program
Washington, DC

Bob Bowen, President
People Directed Supports
Canton, OH

Patsy Buida
Foster Care Specialist
Children's Bureau
Washington, DC

Mary Cesare-Murphy, Ph.D.
Executive Director
Behavioral Health Accreditation
Joint Commission on Accreditation
  of Health Care Organizations
Oakbrook Terrace, IL.

Earl Dunlap, Executive Director
National Juvenile Detention
  Association
Eastern Kentucky University
Richmond, KY

Gary L. Fitzherbert,
Executive Director
Devereux Glenholme School
Washington, CT

Lorraine E. Fox
Training Consultant
Professional Growth Facilitators
San Clemente, CA

Glynn Fraker, RN, M.Ed., CPHQ
Corporate Director of Quality
  Improvement
Devereux Foundation
Villanova, PA

Lindy Garnette, MSW
Director of Children's Primary Care
  Child and Family Mental
  Health Services
National Mental Health Association
Alexandria, VA

Stacey H. Gerber,
Deputy Commissioner
Connecticut Department of
  Children and Families
Hartford, CT

Sharon Gibbons
Child Protective Services
  Coordinator
Washoe County Department of
  Social Services
Reno, NV

Steve Girelli, Ph.D., Vice President
Behavioral Health and Education
Klingberg Family Center, Inc.
New Britain, CT

Saskia Grinberg
Director of Milieu Services
The Home for Little Wanderers
Boston, MA

Richard D. Gritter, President
Wedgewood Christian
  Youth & Family Services
Grand Rapids, MI

Martha Holden, Project Director
Residential Child Care Project
Family Life Development Center
Cornell University
Ithaca, NY

Chris Holloway
Office of Juvenile Justice &
  Delinquency Prevention
Washington, DC

Dr. Anthony Joseph, M.D.
Harvard Medical School
Waltham, MA

Pauline D. Koch, M.S.
Executive Director
National Association for
  Regulatory Administration
Dover, DE

Sherry Kolbe
Executive Director and CEO
National Association of Private
  Special Educational Centers
Washington, DC

Suzanne LeBeau
Director of Training & Compliance
Devereux Massachusetts
Rutland, MA

Robert E. Lieberman, M.A. LPC
President-Elect
American Association of Children's
  Residential Centers
Washington, DC

David H. Mandt, Sr.
President and CEO
David Mandt & Associates
Richardson, TX

Arthur S. Masker
President and CEO
Holston United Methodist
  Home for Children
Greenville, TN

Joy Midman, Executive Director
National Association of Psychiatric
  Treatment Centers for Children
Washington, DC

Andrea Mooney, ESQ
Project Counsel
Cayuga County Safe Schools &
  Healthy Students Partnership, Inc.
Auburn, NY

Joe K. Mullen, Jr.
JKM Training, Inc.
Carlisle, PA

C.T. O'Donnell
President and CEO
Kids Peace National Centers For
  Kids In Crisis
Orefield, PA

Maril Olson, MSW
Director of Child Welfare
Community Education for
  Children's Mental Health
National Mental Health Association
Alexandria, VA

Sil Orlando, Executive Director
Optimist Youth Homes and
  Family Services
Los Angeles, CA

William M. Powers, MPA
Executive Director
The Christie School
Marylhurst, OR

David W. Roush, Ph.D., Director
National Juvenile Detention
  Associations
Center for Research and
  Professional Development
Michigan State University
East Lansing, MI

Randy Ruth, President
National Foster Parent Association
Burnsville, MN

Judith Schubert, Executive Director
Crisis Prevention Institute
Brookfield, WI

Ed Spisszak, R.N., B.A., CPHQ
QA&I Data Analysis
Kids Peace National Center for
  Kids in Crisis
Orefield, PA

Katie McLeese Stephenson, MSW
Family Support Services
  Administrator
Protection and Safety Division
Nebraska Department of Health
  and Human Services
Lincoln, NE

Lawrence D. Swartz
General Counsel
Executive Office of Health &
  Human Services
Boston, MA

Zoe Ann Wignall, Center Director
Children's Home Society of
  Minnesota
St. Paul, MN

APPENDIX B

Best Practice Guidelines Reviewers

Association of Child &
Youth Care Practice (ACYCP)
David Thomas, President
Houston, TX

Bazelon Center for Mental Health
  Law
Laurel Stine, Director of
  Federal Relations
Washington, DC

Black Administration in Child
  Welfare
Child Welfare League of America
  (CWLA)
Washington, DC

Children and Adults with
  Attention-Deficit/Hyperactivity
  Disorder
Clarke Ross, Deputy Executive
Director for Public Policy
Landover, MD

Concord Family and Youth Services
Massachusetts Association of School
  Committees
Robert Gass, CEO
Acton, MA

Council on Accreditation of Services
  for Families and Children, Inc.
Joseph M. Frisino
Director of Standards Development
New York, NY

Federation of Families for
  Children's Mental Health
Trina Osher, Coordinator of
  Public Research
Alexandria, VA

Independent Living Resource Inc.
Bill Griffin, President
Durham, NC

International Association of
  Psychosocial Rehabilitation
  Services
Paul Seifert, Director of
  Government Relations and
  Public Information
Columbia, MD

Joint Commission on Accreditation
  of Health Care Organizations
Mary Cesare-Murphy, Ph.D.
Executive Director
Behavioral Health Accreditation
Oakbrook Terrace, IL

National Advisory Committee
  on Child Day Care
Child Welfare League of America
Washington, DC

National Advisory Committee
  on Foster Care
Child Welfare League of America
Washington, DC

National Advisory Committee
  on Juvenile Justice
Child Welfare League of America
Washington, DC

National Advisory Committee
  on Kinship Care
Child Welfare League of America
Washington, DC

National Advisory Committee
  on Residential Group Care
Child Welfare League of America
Washington, DC

National Alliance for the
  Mentally Ill (NAMI)
Arlington, VA

National Association of
  Black Social Workers
Rudolph C. Smith, President
Detroit, MI

National Association of Protection
  and Advocacy Systems (NAPAS)
Curtis L. Decker, Executive Director
Washington, DC

National Association of State
  Foster Care Managers
Sandra Jackson, Deputy Director
Washington, DC

National Council for Community
  Behavioral Healthcare
Pope Simmons, Senior Vice
  President
Government Relations
Rockville, MD

National Council of Latino
  Executives
Child Welfare League of America
Washington, DC

National Indian Child Welfare
  Association
Terry L. Cross, Executive Director
Portland, OR

National Mental Health Association
Andrea Price, Senior Director
  of Legislative Affairs
Alexandria, VA

National Organization of State
  Associations for Children
  (NOSAC)
James P. McComb,
Executive Director
Arnold, MD

SCAR/Jasper Mountain
Dave Ziegler, Executive Director
Jasper, OR.

Senator Christopher Dodd
U. S. Senate

Jim Fenton, Professional Staff
Children and Families
  Subcommittee
Subcommittee on Health,
  Education, Labor, and Pensions
Washington, DC

University of Pittsburgh
School of Social Work
Martha Mattingly, Ph.D
Pittsburgh, PA

Glossary

Administration   The persons who are responsible for the provider's management functions, including fiscal and personnel resources, and ser-vice delivery. Such persons determine provider goals, acquire and allocate resources to carry out a program, coordinate activities toward goal achievement, and monitor, evaluate, and make needed changes in processes and procedures to improve the likelihood of goal achievement.

Admission   The child or youth's physical entry into or arrival at the provider's facility or program.

Agency   An entity with an administrative structure, most often a government, child placing, or regulatory entity.

Behavior Management   The use of specialized interventions to guide, redirect, modify, or manage behavior of children and youth. Behavior management includes a wide range of actions and interventions used in a broad continuum of settings in which adults are responsible for the care and safety of children and youth. These settings include, but are not limited to, residential group care, family foster care, psychiatric hospitals, day treatment, child day care and school-age child care, in-home services, educational programs, shelter care, and juvenile detention. Behavior management includes the entire spectrum of activities from preventative and planned use of the environment, routines, and structure of the particular setting; to less restrictive interventions such as positive reinforcement, verbal interventions, deescalation techniques, therapeutic activities, loss of privileges; to more restrictive interventions such as time-out, physical escorts, physical/chemical/mechanical restraints, and seclusion.

Best Practice   Recommended services, supports, interventions, policies or procedures based upon current validated research and/or expert consensus.

Caregiver   Any individual who provides direct services to children and youth. Caregivers may work independently, as in the case of foster homes or family child care homes, or they may be employees of larger providers.

Family The parent(s) of the child or youth, or the person(s) performing the parental role. Family may include birth or adoptive parents, grandparents, siblings, foster parents, legal guardians, or any other person in a parental role.

Intake The process during which a child or youth's eligibility to receive services is assessed in comparison to the provider's established criteria.

Least Restrictive The settings and interventions that most closely meet the needs of individuals, while most closely approximating the situations of persons who do not need such settings and interventions.

Physical Escort The temporary touching or holding of the hand, wrist, arm, shoulder, or back for the purpose of inducing an individual to walk to a safe location.

Policies Written requirements that direct the business and service-delivery practices within the provider agency. They should carry the approval of the provider's governing or advisory board.

Procedures Written guidelines developed by the provider's administration to ensure that provider practice is consistent with board-approved policies.

Provider Any facility, organization, agency, institution, program, or person that provides services to children and adolescents. In general, provider means the organization, while caregiver refers to an individual. In some settings, the provider and caregiver may be a single person.

Restraint, Chemical The use of any psychoactive medication as a restraint to control behavior or restrict the individual's freedom of movement that is not a standard treatment for the individual's medical or psychiatric condition.

Restraint, Mechanical The use of any physical device to limit movement and prevent harm to self or others. Mechanical restraint does not include devices such as orthopedically prescribed devices, surgical dressings or bandages, protective helmets, or any other methods that involve the physical holding of a resident for the purpose of conducting routine physical examination or tests, or to protect the resident from falling out of bed, or to permit the resident to participate in activities without the risk of physical harm to the resident.

Restraint, Physical The application of physical force by one or more individuals that reduces or restricts the ability of an individual to move his or her arms, legs, or head freely. Physical restraint does not include the temporary physical holding of an individual to permit the individual to participate in activities of daily living (ADL) without the risk of physical harm to the individual.

Restraint-Associated Asphyxia A lack of oxygen caused by interruption in breathing and causing unconsciousness that occurs during or as a result of restraint. Restraint-associated asphyxia may lead to death.

Restrictive Behavior Management Interventions Interventions that restrict, limit, or curtail an individual's freedom of movement to prevent harm to self or others. Restrictive interventions include, but are not limited to physical, mechanical, and chemical restraint, and seclusion.

Seclusion The placement of an individual against his or her will in any room where the door is unable to be opened voluntarily by the individual, in order to prevent harm to self or others.

Service Plan A written plan of action that identifies needs, sets goals, and describes strategies and timelines for achieving goals.

Staff A person or persons who are employed by the provider in any role including administrative, management, supervisory, or caregiving.

Targeted Behavior A behavior identified in a child or youth's individualized service plan as the behavior needing to be modified or eliminated. Targeted behavior(s) should be observable and measurable.

Therapeutic Hold A physical restraint.

Time-Out A procedure in which an individual is not given the opportunity to receive positive reinforcement and/or participation in the current routine or activity is suspended for specific behavior(s). The length of the time-out interval should be short and based on the individual's developmental level, limited to the period necessary for the individual to calm down. The criteria for ending the time-out should be communicated to the individual.

Nonexclusionary Time-Out Separation of an individual from a group or activity in a manner that prevents reinforcement, but still allows the individual the opportunity to observe others participating in appropriate behavior and receiving positive reinforcement. When non-exclusionary time-out is used, the individual is not removed from the environment.

Exclusionary Time-Out Removal of an individual from a reinforcing activity to a specified location where he or she is unable to participate or observe the activity, either visually or audibly. The specified location must be an area that does not contain any mechanical and/or physical barriers that prevent an individual from leaving voluntarily.

Selected References

Academy for Youth Development, Center for Youth Development and Policy Research (1996, April). *Best practices in community based youth worker training.* Washington, DC: Author.

Alwon, F. J. (2000). *Effective supervisory practice: A confidence building curriculum for supervisors and managers (Parts I & II, Instructor's Guides).* Washington, DC: CWLA Press.

Alwon, F. J., Blome, W. W., & Lutz, R. M. (1999). Whatever the problem, the answer is training—Or is it? *Common Ground, 16*(1), 8–9.

Alwon, F. J., & Reitz, A. L. (2000). *The workforce crisis in child welfare: An issue brief.* Washington, DC: CWLA Press.

American Academy of Pediatrics (1995). Informed consent, parental permission, and assent in pediatric practice (RE9510). *Policy Statement, 95,* 2.

American Academy of Pediatrics and American Public Health Association (in print). *Caring for our children—National health and safety performance standards: Guidelines for out-of-home child care* (2nd ed.). Washington, DC: Author.

Buckinham, M., & Coffman, C. (1999). *First, break all the rules: What the world's greatest managers do differently.* New York: Simon & Schuster.

Council on Accreditation for Children and Family Services. (2001). *Standards and self study manual* (7th ed.). New York: Author.

Draves, W. A. (1984). *How to teach adults.* Manhattan, KS: Learning Resources Network.

Hyson, M. C. (2000). *Research document for revision of Delacare: Requirements for child care centers.* Newark: University of Delaware.

Joint Commission on Accreditation of Healthcare Organizations (2001). *2001–2002 Standards for behavioral health care.* Oakbrook Terrace, IL: Joint Commission Resources.

Krueger, M. (1998). *Interactive youth work practice.* Washington, DC: CWLA Press.

Mattingly, M. (in press). *Proposed competencies for professional child and youth work personnel.* Milwaukee, WI: Association for Child and Youth Care Practice.

National Association for the Education of Young Children. (1997). *Guide to accreditation by the National Association for the Education of Young Children.* Washington, DC: National Academy of Early Childhood Programs.

National Association for Regulatory Administration. http://www.nara-licensing.org/

North American Consortium of Child and Youth Care Education Programs (1995). Special report: Curriculum content for child and youth care practice. *Child and Youth Care Forum, 23*(4), 269–278.

Reitz, A.L. (1998). *Child and youth worker core training course (unpublished curriculum).* Washington, DC: Child Welfare League of America.

Rosenberg, D. (2000). *A manager's guide to hiring the best person for every job.* New York: John Wiley & Sons.

Shield, J. P. H., & Baum, J. D. (1994, May). Children's consent to treatment. *British Medical Journal, 308,* 1182–83.

Siegfried, C. (1999). *Checking up on juvenile justice facilities: A handbook for child mental health advocates.* Alexandria, VA: National Mental Health Association.

Small, R. W., & Dodge, L. M. (1988). Roles, skills, and job tasks in professional child care: A review of the literature. *Child and Youth Care Quarterly, 17*(1), 6–21.

Stein, Thedore J. (1998). *Child welfare and the law.* Washington, DC: CWLA Press.

Trieschman, A. E., Whittaker, J. K., & Brendto, L. K. (1969). *The other 23 hours: Child-care work with emotionally disturbed children in a therapeutic milieu.* New York: Aldine de Gruyter.

U. S. Department of Health and Human Services, Healthcare Financing Administration. (2001). *Safeguarding Medicaid's younger persons with serious mental illnesses.* HHS News Press Release. Washington, DC: Health Care Financing Administration, Press Office.

VanderVen, K. (1998). *Dimensions of a milieu.* Handout packet for activity programming workshops. Pittsburgh, PA.

VanderVen, K. (1998). *Some working principles of activity programming.* Handout packet for activity programming workshops. Pittsburgh, PA.

VanderVen, K. (1998). *A balanced developmental/therapeutic activity program.* Handout packet for activity programming workshops. Pittsburgh, PA.

VanderVen, K. (1999). You are what you do and become what you've done. *Journal of Child and Youth Care, 18*(2), 133–147.

Wheatley, M. (1999). *Leadership and the new science* (2nd ed.). San Francisco: Berrett-Koehler.

Selected Additional Resources

American Academy of Physician Assistants website: www.aapa.org/gandp/restraint.html.

American Association of Children's Residential Centers (2000). *Position paper on restraint and seclusion.* Washington, DC: Author.

American Correctional Association website: www.corrections.com/aca.

American Medical Association. (n.d.). *Report 10 of the Council on Scientific Affairs (A-99).* www.ama-assn.org/ama/pub/article/2036-2339.html.

American Psychological Association, Commission of Violence and Youth (1993). *Violence and youth: Psychology's response* (Vol. 1). Washington, DC: Author.

Anderson, J. (1990). *Holding therapy: A way of helping unattached children.* In Grabe (Ed.), Adoption resources for mental health professionals. Piscataway, NJ:Transaction Publishers.

Aschen, S. R. (1995). Restraints: Does position make a difference? *Issues in Mental Health Nursing 16*(1), 87–92.

Bath, H. (1994). The physical restraint of children—Is it therapeutic? *The American Journal of Orthopsychiatry, 64*(1).

Brooks, K. L., Mulaik, J. S., et al. (1994). Patient overcrowding in psychiatric hospital units: Effects on seclusion and restraint. *Administration and Policy in Mental Health 22*(3), 133–134.

Fassler, D., & Cotton, N. (1992). A national survey on the use of seclusion in the psychiatric hospitalization of children. *Hospital and Community Psychiatry, 43*(4).

Fisher, W. (1994). Restraint and seclusion: A review of the literature. *American Journal of Psychiatry, 151*(11).

Garrison, W. (1984). Inpatient psychiatric treatment of the difficult child: Common practices and their ethical implications. *Children and Youth Services Review, 6.*

Goren, S., Singh, N., & Best, A. M. (1993). The aggression-coercion cycle: Use of seclusion and restraint in a child psychiatric hospital. *Journal of Child & Family Studies, 2*(1).

Gunn, S. (2000, May). *Organizational systems to minimize restraint and maximize dignity, effective treatment, and safety.* Paper presented at the Walker Trieschman Center's Finding Better Ways Conference.

Hanson, R., (Ed.). (1982). *Institutional abuse of children and youth.* New York: Haworth Press.

Holden, M., et al. (2001). *Therapeutic crisis intervention: A train the trainer curriculum.* Ithaca, NY: Family Development Center.

Holden, M. J., & Powers, J. L. (1993). Therapeutic crisis intervention. *Journal of Emotional and Behavioral Problems 2*(1).

Howells, K. & Hollin, C. R. (1989). *Clinical approaches to violence.* New York: John Wiley and Sons.

Irwin, M. (1987). Are seclusion rooms needed on child psychiatric units? *American Journal of Orthopsychiatry, 57.*

Levy, T. M., & Orlans, M. (1998). *Attachment, trauma, and healing: Understanding and treating attachment disorder in children and families.* Washington, DC: CWLA Press.

Mohr, W. (1998). A restraint on restraint: The need to consider restrictive interventions. *Archives of Psychiatric Nursing, 12*(2).

National Alliance for the Mentally Ill website: www.nami.org/update/ unitedrestraint.html.

National Association of Psychiatric Health Services website: www.naphs.org/ News/ guidingprinc.html.

New York State Coalition for Children's Mental Health Services. (2001). *Survey on the use of Physical Holds, Albany, NY.* Unpublished raw data.

Ray, N., & Myers, K. (1996). Patient perspectives on restraint and seclusion experiences: A survey of former patients of New York state psychiatric facilities. *Psychiatric Rehabilitation Journal, 20*(1).

Rich, C. (1997). The use of physical restraint in residential treatment: An ego psychology perspective. *Residential Treatment for Children and Youth, 14*(3).

Rindfleisch, N. (1978). A study of the influence of background and organizational factors on direct care worker's attitudes toward the use of physical force on children. *Dissertation Abstracts, 38*(3). (See R. Hanson (1982), *Institutional abuse of children and youth,* pp. 115–125.)

Singh, N. (1997). *Prevention and treatment of severe behavioral problems: Models and methods in developmental disabilities.* Pacific Grove, CA: Brooks-Cole Publishing.

Tobin, L. (1991). *What do you do with a child like this: Inside the lives of troubled children.* Duluth, MN: Whole Person Associates.

Trieschman, A. E., Whittaker, J. K., & Brendto, L. K. (1969). *The Other 23 Hours: Child-care work with emotionally disturbed children in a therapeutic milieu.* New York: Aldine de Gruyter.

Tsemberis, S., & Sullivan, C. (1988). Seclusion in context: Introducing a seclusion room into a children's unit of a municipal hospital. *American Journal of Orthopsychiatry, 58*(3).

Turnbull, J., & Patterson, B. (1999). *Aggression and violence: Approaches to effective management.* London, UK: MacMillan Press, Ltd.